RAW FOOD

Your Guide & Cookbook to a Healthy Raw Food Diet

Written By

Body and Soul Mastery

monetary loss due to the information herein, either directly or indirectly.

Respective authors own all copyrights not held by the publisher.

The information herein is offered for informational purposes solely, and is universal as so. The presentation of the information is without contract or any type of guarantee assurance.

The trademarks that are used are without any consent, and the publication of the trademark is without permission or backing by the trademark owner. All trademarks and brands within this book are for clarifying purposes only and are the owned by the owners themselves, not affiliated with this document.

Table of Contents

Introduction

I want to thank you and congratulate you for downloading the book, "Raw Food Diet 101 - Beginners Guide and Introduction to Raw Food Diet".

We all desire to live healthier more productive lives and well, most of the foods we eat are highly processed, high in sugar, unhealthy fats and salts. Because of consumption of such kinds of foods, we end up gaining weight, suffering from lifestyle diseases like high blood pressure, diabetes and heart diseases and we end up depriving our bodies of essential nutrients.

The truth is that most diets out there are quite restrictive, which can lead to your body lacking certain nutrients. This then leads to cravings, and the cycle continues. The thing about a raw food diet is that it will not only help you lose weight but you will also be providing your body with essential nutrients since the nutrients have not been damaged by heat.

I know most people think that the only raw thing you can have for breakfast is a smoothie and a salad. Well, I will prove you wrong because I will provide you with some amazing raw pancakes, raw bread and raw bagels recipes to get you started on your raw food diet journey. You will not only enjoy being on this diet but you will also lose weight and have more energy, which will also make you more productive.

If getting a new variety of raw foods will make you stick to your raw food diet plan, this book is all you need to begin your healthy journey and ENJOY your new Breakfast, Lunch, and Dinner Menus right at home.!

This book has a wide array of different recipes that you can try today; from the salads and soups to amazing ceviche and beef tartare. With these recipes, you are bound to have an amazing time on a raw food diet.

Thanks again for downloading this book, I hope you enjoy it!

Spiralizer with a Twist

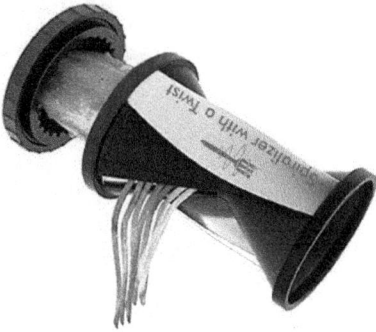

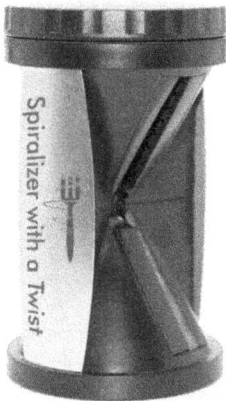

Click below to get this amazing kitchen tool, that can help create some of these delicious meals.

http://amzn.to/1M21yjt

Are you aware that food is the healthiest and most nutritious when consumed uncooked? This is because when you don't cook, you conserve the enzymes that help in both absorption and digestion of food. On the other hand, cooking kills or denatures these enzymes. For instance, the cancer fighting sulforaphanes found in broccoli are denatured after cooking. In addition, most of the vitamin C and folate found in veggies is destroyed by cooking. However, the fibrous portion in some foods may increase after cooking. For instance, cooked tomatoes can have 3-4 times more lycopene as compared to raw tomatoes. That notwithstanding, eating raw seeds, nuts, veggies and unprocessed natural fruits offers more nutrients and vitamins and facilitates the detox process in the body. I am sure you would want to know how you stand to benefit by embracing a raw food diet. So to get started, we will start our beginner's guide to a raw food diet with the benefits you stand to gain by eating raw food.

Benefits Of Being On A Raw Food Diet

Though scientific research doesn't necessarily approve the diet to cure certain health conditions, those on the diet have indicated being healed of various ailments as well as having more energy while on a raw food diet. We will look at some of the benefits that you stand to gain while on a raw food diet. Some of these benefits include:

- Weight loss

When on a raw food diet, you eat more of vegetables, seeds, fruits, nuts, some legumes, and healthy fats and oils, which all enhance satiety. This means you will be consuming less food because you will be becoming fuller quickly. In addition, enzymes found in raw food facilitate weight loss. Some of these enzymes include lipase, an enzyme that helps breakdown fats thus helping in the digestion of fats and thus its breakdown to produce energy.

- Reduced risk of diseases

Raw food has little trans-fats and saturated fats as well as very low in sugar and sodium. It is however rich in fiber, folate, magnesium and potassium, vitamin A and other antioxidants that promote good health. Such minerals and

10

nutrients also assist in fighting diseases such as cancer, diabetes, and heart disease. Raw food has also been proven to lower total cholesterol and triglyceride levels in the blood plasma.

Raw food is also perfect for its acid-alkaline balance. In addition, since raw food has low advanced glycation end products, it can help reduce inflammation.

- You get more phytonutrients, vitamins & minerals

Phytonutrients are the important antioxidants that you obtain from fruits and veggies, useful in fighting chronic diseases like cancer. They activate your metabolism at a cellular level and monitor hormones that help in controlling appetite. Cooking usually destroys majority of phytonutrients and vitamins thus translates to eating 'empty foods' with insufficient beneficial compounds for your cells.

- Intake of more enzymes, which help in digestion and boosting energy

Enzymes are required in most body processes and help in digestion of raw or cooked food. Actually, eating of an enzyme-rich diet has shown to boost vitality and slow down the aging process, as enzymes are involved in repair of DNA and RNA. For instance, protease enzyme helps break down proteins into amino acids or the body's building blocks and helps remove toxins from the body.

These enzymes are killed by heat above 118 degrees F.

•   Increased intake of quality proteins

A plant-based diet has higher quality of proteins and is easier to digest and absorb into the cells, as the protein is found in cells whose walls are made of fiber. Fiber usually facilitates digestion, and lacks in animal-based proteins. Furthermore, animal cells are made of cholesterol, which the body doesn't break down easily, and can lead to constipation.

Raw food diet incorporates majority of plant proteins and greens, thus you're able to obtain the 8 essential amino acids required by cells.

One of the major benefits of a raw food diet is that it helps balance your body pH. Let us look closely at raw food and its role in pH of your bloodstream.

Raw Food Diet pH

I am sure you have come across the word "pH balance", which is very important for good health. PH balance simply means the balance between alkalinity and acidity. Most of us can remember the science experiments we did in school when determining if something is alkaline or acidic using strips of litmus paper. We were basically measuring substances' "potential for Hydrogen", which then indicates if a substance has more alkaline or acidic molecules. A pH of 7 is neutral, above 7 is alkaline and below 7 is acidic.

In order for your body to function adequately, the bloodstream ought to be slightly alkaline with a pH of 7.4. Since the blood usually provides all the necessary nutrients, when it is too acidic, it can harm the internal organs and cause a state of imbalance. Additionally, majority of body enzymes work in alkaline conditions.

If the blood pH goes below 7.35, you will suffer from a condition known as acidosis, which can cause chronic illness, headaches, body odor, and slower rate of enzymatic reactions that inhibit the production of energy from glucose as well as synthesis of proteins or vitamins. In addition, in acidic conditions, the body utilizes minerals in its stores when trying to combat the acidity. This effect has a negative impact on bones and teeth that are mainly composed of minerals, thus conditions like osteoporosis and dental problems often develops.

So how does a raw food diet help you? In most cases, our blood can become too acidic due to our lifestyle choices. Some of the acidic foods include:

• Saturated fats

• Dairy products such as butter, cheese and milk

• Peas and cashews

• Grains among them bread, flour, pasta, rice, and white wheat

• Most animal foods as oysters, fish, chicken, eggs and meat

• Sugar and highly processed foods

Therefore, embracing a raw food diet can be your ticket to achieving pH balance. This is because these foods increase the oxygen content that your blood absorbs, most of them being raw green leafy veggies, non-sweet grasses and fruits. Some alkaline foods include:

• Sprouts such as broccoli, mung beans and alfalfa

• Wheat grass

• Fruits such as young coconuts, cucumber, avocado, watermelon

• Fresh herbs and spices e.g. ginger, cayenne, cilantro, basil, parsley

• Veggies particularly leafy green vegetables

• Alkaline drinks like wheatgrass juice, vegetable juice, and young coconut water.

Basically, consuming of raw fresh fruits, veggies and their juices plays an important role in balancing the pH of your body. You should thus add dark leafy greens to juices and smoothies, alongside other variety of fresh fruits and veggies, nuts and seeds. Herbal sweeteners like stevia also serve to alkalinize the body and boost enzymatic reactions.

Basic Cleansing Raw Food

One other benefit of eating raw food is raw foods' ability to detox and cleanse your body. Eating raw food helps eliminate toxins and other contaminants in your cells and body fat. This leads to improved health, more energy, better digestion, and an improved memory and immune system. However, it's important to ensure your body has alkaline minerals that facilitate detox. You will need minerals like iron, sodium, phosphorous, sulfur, magnesium and calcium, otherwise your cells may fail to release the toxins stored as body fat. Such toxins are then reabsorbed into the body again and interfere with metabolic activities.

Before a detox diet, alkalinize by eating a lot of green veggies and fresh fruits. For instance, try adding wheatgrass powder or blue green algae into your smoothie or pure water to obtain minerals and amino acids. Also, drink fruit juices, green vegetable juice and water to help eliminate waste. Below are some amazing food that when taken raw can help detox your body:

Fruits

Go for fresh and organic varieties of fruits such as prunes, raisins, apricots, peaches, pear, blackberry, blueberry, raspberry, strawberry, watermelon, cantaloupe, lime, lemon, grape fruit, orange, kiwi, papaya, pineapple, mango, grapes, banana and apple.

Vegetables

Opt for both green leafy vegetables and starchy vegetables like seaweed, squash, zucchini, asparagus, watercress, celery, parsley, garlic, ginger, green onion, onion, peppers, carrots, cabbage, broccoli, kales, spinach, dark green or red lettuce etc

Seeds

Try raw seeds such as pumpkin, chia, hemp, flax, and sunflower

Nuts

Best raw nuts include macadamia, pine nuts, pistachio, walnuts, cashew, and almonds

Legumes

Legumes to eat on detox include raw bean sprouts, edamame, lentils, kidney beans, mung beans and chickpeas.

Unprocessed grains

Reach for raw varieties of unprocessed bulgur, millet, quinoa, buckwheat, granola, oats and other whole grain cereals.

Other foods

In addition to these raw foods, include various herbs and spices, raw cocoa powder, raw protein powder, almond and nut butters, raw and unfiltered vinegar as well as raw extra-virgin olive and coconut oils.

Drinks

You can drink a variety of substances ranging from non-dairy milk such as soy or almond milk, herbal teas, coconut water, fresh juices, unsweetened drinks, filtered water and vegetable smoothies among others.

Let us now have a look at foods that you will be eating while on a raw food diet.

Basic Raw Food Proteins

On a raw diet, you can obtain your proteins from leafy greens and sprouts, which are high in protein. Other sources of proteins include legumes, nuts, seeds, and grains. The following are some of the richest source of proteins on a raw food diet:

Fruit

Fruits contains around 5-10 percent protein with all the 8 essential amino acids your body requires to build new body cells. If you consume about 18-22 grams of proteins from fruits daily, you have obtained half of your daily protein content. Apart from ordinary fruits like berries and apples, reach for non-sweet fruits such as cucumber, and tomatoes.

Leafy Green Vegetables

Leafy green vegetables are rich in proteins, with 2 large bunches of dark leafy greens offering 14-20 grams of protein. For instance, a head of lettuce should give you 5 grams of proteins, while 2 cups of kales offer 4 grams of proteins. You can take the veggies by shredding them or making green smoothies. Other amazing sources of protein include parsley, broccoli, spinach, celery, and artichokes.

Nuts & Seeds

19

These are rich in proteins and you can take them as regular snacks. Try Brazilian nuts and seeds such as pumpkin as they are very high in protein. Additionally, an ounce of cashew nuts should provide around 5 grams of proteins with chia seeds yielding 4.4 grams. A tablespoon of flaxseeds has about 2 grams while ¼ cup of sunflower seeds has 7.3 grams of proteins. Try carrying a few hemp and flax seeds and snack on them whenever hungry to energize and fuel your cells.

Protein Powders

It's advisable to incorporate protein powders when transiting to a raw diet to help your body obtain this essential nutrient as you adapt. Powders from sprouted protein are the best since they are made from gluten free, raw protein and vegan source. Protein powder such as Sprout Living and Epic Protein has about 23 grams of proteins, and blends well in smoothies without a chalky texture found in some protein powders. They also come in various flavors.

Other protein sources you should try out are;

-The blue-green algae also known as spirulina

-Sprouted grains such as wild rice and quinoa

-Sprouted lentils

-Sprouted beans such as garbanzo, chick peas and mung beans

-Mushrooms such as portabella, shiitake and cremini

Basic Raw Food Carbs

Carbs are an important part of the diet, as they facilitate the functioning of cells while offering energy to fuel metabolic activities. While on a raw diet, you can get carbs from starchy veggies, cereal grain and legumes.

Starchy Vegetables

These include veggies such as pumpkin, artichokes, cassava root, caladium root, yams, and water squashes such as banana and buttercup squashes. Other mild starchy vegetables include salsify, rutabaga, cauliflower and carrots.

Cereal grains

Cereals should be whole and unrefined, such as oats, rye, millet, wheat, or barley.

Legumes

These include the beans, peas, peanuts, and lentils that can be consumed raw such as mung beans.

Fruits

Sweet fruits and non-sweet fruits such as tomatoes, cucumbers, squashes, and bell peppers can also serve as source of carbohydrates while on a raw food diet. Sweet fruits such as grapefruits and cranberry are rich in sugar, which serves as source of energy for body cells. Avoid green peppers or those fruits without seeds like seedless grapes.

You can also have dried fruits. These include dried apples, mangoes, apricot, coconut, pineapple, goji berries, cranberries, raisins and dates. Dates serves as preferable sweeteners especially for raw food deserts.

Basic Raw Food Fats

The best sources of fats while on a raw diet are durians, coconuts, olives, avocado, nuts and seeds. The body requires fats and oils as they are filling and satisfy hunger without need to overeat. Fats also help feed nerves and thus reduce stress while keeping you healthy. It's advisable to soak your olives for a few hours to remove the excess salt or marinate fresh herbs into some olive oil for extra deliciousness. Choose raw and unrefined nut and seed oils, which have been cold pressed at low temperature to avoid free radical damage or oxidation.

A number of seeds and nuts are rich in omega 3 fatty acids among them hemp, walnuts, flax and their respective oils. You can also get omega 6 fatty acids from nuts, seeds, seed oils, nut oils, hempseed oil, and borage oil. Try to avoid saturated fats, animal proteins, cholesterol, trans-fatty acids and refined carbs. Fats from these sources often trigger an inflammatory response and lead to chronic diseases. So how can you incorporate these healthy fats and oils

*Avocados: Try incorporating them into salads, blend them into green soup or guacamole, mash them up and toss with cacao powder or soaked dates into a blender to make a pudding.

*For healthy oils and fats, use unheated oils in dips, green soups, salads, and smoothies

*You can utilize nuts and seeds with their milk such as nut milk. To make nut milk, just soak 1 part seeds in 3 parts water for a few hours or overnight, strain through a nut milk bag and obtain your milk. You can use nut milk in smoothies, cereals, salads among others. Nut and seed butters are useful when topping crackers, fruits and veggies.

*Coconut: This serves as a good fat source and can be used in smoothies and other foods. You can add shredded coconut to cacao or avocado pudding or use coconut butter.

Now that we have looked at what you can eat, let us have a look at what is not advisable to eat. It is important to understand most people simply think that while on a raw food diet, you simply eat anything without having to cook. This is however not the case because some foods even vegetables may not be advisable to eat hence we will look at what you should not eat while on a raw food diet.

What Not To Eat

In addition to not eating cooked foods while on a raw food diet, you also need to avoid some foods that are considered unsafe among them beans. Avoid beans such as fava beans, soybeans and kidney beans. However, you might eat some beans but ensure they are first soaked and sprouted. Also avoid consuming foods that are grown using pesticides, or with added food colors, dyes, preservatives or other additives. Among those foods you shouldn't eat on raw food diet includes:

• Parsnips: They have a chemical referred to as furanocoumarin, basically produced by the plant as a self defense against predators. These chemicals are toxic to the human metabolic system.

• Cassava and cassava flour: This is because most varieties are toxic

• Peas: Raw peas such as glass pea can lead to neurological weakness of the lower limb, a condition known as lathyrism.

• Buckwheat greens: The greens are poisonous when consumed raw. Furthermore, buckwheat can also be poisonous if juiced or if eaten in plenty as it triggers skin problems or photosensitivity.

26

- Kidney beans: Raw kidney beans and its sprouts are toxic due to presence of a chemical referred to as phytohaemagglutinin.

- Raw eggs: Raw eggs contain a poisonous substance referred to as avadin. Consuming up to 24 raw eggs has been found to interfere with utilization of vitamin B7 in the body. Additionally, some raw eggs have salmonella bacteria, which medics say might cause serious illness when eggs aren't cooked.

- Apricot kernels: These have a poisonous chemical called amygdalin

- Raw meat: Raw meat may have dangerous viruses, parasites and bacteria.

- Alfalfa sprouts: These have a poisonous chemical called canavanine

- Taro

- Rhubarb leaves

- Potatoes

How To Prepare Raw Food

Well, now that you understand what to eat and what to avoid, the next thing is to understand how to prepare the foods without cooking. Let us look at how to prepare raw food.

Soaking and Sprouting

Raw foods such are seeds, nuts, legumes and beans have enzyme inhibitors that are denatured through cooking. To help release the nutrients in the highest concentration, you can soak, germinate, or sprout them. For germination, soak the food in water for a certain period of time say 2 hours or 1 day for mung beans. For better results, soak your food overnight. In order to soak the seeds, nuts or legumes:

-First rinse the seeds, legumes, nuts, or beans and then put them in a glass container.

-Add water at room temperature to cover and soak the food preferably overnight.

-After soaking for at least 2 hours, rinse them a number of times and then use.

For sprouting, you proceed after germination. You drain your legumes, beans, and seeds during the last step of germination and then put them in a different container to sprout. Leave them until they open and a sprout starts to grow then rinse the sprouted seeds or nuts and then drain them. Store the sprouted food in an airtight container in the fridge for around 5 days.

Dehydrating

Here you can put the food under temperatures lower than 118 degrees F, in a dehydrator to facilitate sun drying. A dehydrator is an enclosed container that has heating elements that warm the food at low temperatures. It has a fan that blows warm air into the food placed spread out on trays. Such equipment can be used to prepare fruit leathers, croutons, breads, crackers, kale chips, sundried tomatoes, and raisins.

Blending

This is the easiest method of preparing raw food. Blending is preferred to make recipes for soups, smoothies, humus ad pesto.

Other methods of preparing raw foods include:

• Juicing

• Pickling

• Fermenting: For instance, preparing sauerkraut to have a tasty spice for other raw foods

You should also have some essential equipment to prepare raw food in addition to a dehydrator. They include:

1. Spiral slicer to help cut your veggies into spiral shapes

2. Containers to sprout or mason jars

3. Trays or large containers to soak or germinate seeds, beans, and grains

4. Food processor or blender to prepare nut milks, soups, and smoothies

5. A thermometer to ensure that the temperatures remain at 118F inside the dehydrator

6. Juicers to help you adopt more fruits and veggies into your diet. However, be aware eating raw fruit is healthier than juicing since the juices don't have fiber while eating the whole fruit will ensure you get some fiber.

9. Solar oven, which utilizes low heat to preserve the desired nutrients. You can use the solar oven in multiple dishes to prepare patties, crackers, dips, cold or hot soups.

Now that you know what to eat, the foods to avoid as well as how to prepare these foods, let us now look at how you can get started on a raw food diet.

How to Get Started on a Raw Food Diet

1. Consider the source of your food

As you switch to raw food, ensure that you get products from credible sources free from chemicals used in conventional farming. Chemicals are harmful for your body and environment. To avoid eating food grow with chemical pesticides, fertilizers and other addictives, try the following:

-Grow your own food. You should try different sprouts and herbs, where you can even grow veggies from a sunny windowsill to ensure you get healthy crops all year round.

-Prepare your own compost to ensure the nutritional content of food is higher. You can use a worm composter or ordinary compost bin

-Ensure that you purchase organic products from credible sources. In case you find the price too high, only buy those foods highly recommended or basic food to eat on a raw healthy diet.

You need to do thorough research on where crops are grown from as some crops are heavily sprayed or intensively raised compared to others. Thus, it might be advisable to buy organic produce straight from the farms where you can follow through on how the crops are raised.

2. Stock up your kitchen gradually

Having sufficient choices of foods is important when transitioning to a raw food diet to ensure you get a variety of tastes. Ensure that you buy enough supply of fresh whole foods, fruits and veggies, where you can gradually increase the supply of these foods in your fridge or kitchen shelve.

Buy enough dried herbs such as dill, rosemary, thyme, oregano, basil among others.

-You also need spices such as black pepper, cayenne powder, turmeric powder, onion powder, garlic powder, coriander powder, nutmeg powder, cumin powder, and cinnamon.

-Get adequate nuts among them macadamia, pecans, hazel nuts, walnuts, pine nuts, cashew nuts and almonds

-Incorporate seeds into your raw diet like sesame seeds, chia seeds, flaxseeds, pumpkin seeds, sunflower seeds and others

-You should also stock on oils and butters like cold-pressed olive oil, flaxseed oil, virgin coconut oil, nut butter and raw organic cacao butter.

-Buy organic sweeteners such as raw honey, organic coconut palm nectar, stevia, and natural flavor enhancer such as tamari, sea salt, and miso.

These raw and organic ingredients are important when preparing raw foods or desserts.

3. Learn how to prepare raw food

Common food preparation methods practiced by most people include boiling, grilling, frying, steaming, baking, braising among others. These methods all involve heating of food to extreme temperatures, which kills important enzymes. Raw foods on the other hand shouldn't be heated to over 48°C, thus you'll need to use methods such as blending, dehydrating, fermenting, grating, sprouting, marinating, juicing, culturing, pickling, soaking and grinding.

With research and patience, you can learn other ways of incorporating various flavors, such as using different ingredients to balance flavor. You should also take fats since they are important in making the food have a cooked texture. Research can help you learn about the raw binders or thickening agents alongside the substitutes you can use for raw ingredients.

4. Plan your meals

Try preparing your food ingredients earlier before you get to finish organizing a whole raw dish. For instance, you might try to soak the nuts, or prepare the nut cheese and pesto in advance before you make the raw pizza. Also, try to make the chocolate drizzle in advance to later incorporate to your chocolate and save time. Though this might seem difficult or complicated for beginners, the basics involve deciding your recipes, grouping the ingredients based on their preparation time, and preparing those requiring more time in advance. You can also deal with ingredients that require separate preparation and later assemble everything together.

You also need to plan for possible substitutions for snacks or treats by having enough bites at coffee time or midnight. Ensure that you plan for your entire day or week's supply of crackers to avoid eating sugary and unhealthy foods. Dehydrated fruit slices and flaxseeds crackers make a good choice. Just make it your custom to plan and include various raw snack recipes into your kitchen schedule.

5. Start small with easy to make recipes

Begin with those simple meals that require locally available ingredients from supermarkets, groceries, or local markets. If you find it hard to switch to 100 percent raw food, try to include a few raw ingredients into the diet for a start. Get variety of foods by making a list of nuts and seeds, herbs or other ingredients to form part of your diet. For instance, start with fresh fruits for breakfast or an alternative fresh fruit smoothie each breakfast without dairy.

Then adopt the rest of raw food into your diet on a weekly basis, by eating a salad for lunch and dinner, alongside sprouted beans, sprouted seeds, nuts and other seeds. Use fresh herbs, non-dairy seasonings, raw food plant-based pates and other ingredients. Try adding hummus in various meals, as flavors make raw food edible, while herbs make salads tasty. Adopt the accepted methods of preparing food and learn how to prepare desserts to ensure you don't forsake your sweet tooth, since depriving yourself of things you love can easily lead to cravings.

6. Know how to store foods properly

Be aware that raw food is prone to damage and cannot keep long compared to processed food. Eat your raw food within few days of purchase as you replenish them often. Ensure you consume food within the set time for use, bearing in mind their quality deteriorates with time. For homegrown crops, harvest them only when needed, to ensure freshness during use. Food ingredients such as grains, coconut, carob, dried fruits, nuts, and seeds can be stored under refrigeration for a longer period.

7. Ensure that you blend drinks as opposed to juicing as blended drinks have high fiber content.

8. To prevent problems such as anemia, ensure you supplement with vitamin B12.

9. You might carry your own ingredients into restaurants or other dinning places such as herbs, natural salad dressing, lemon, and avocado. Ask ahead if such practice is acceptable

or if such products are served as part of the diet. If such arrangement does not exist, you can order a salad and later eat other foods at home.

10. For animal products, be cautious of their quality and source to ensure they have been raised organically and free form harsh chemicals.

Precautions In Eating Raw Food

Despite the amazing benefits you stand to benefit by adapting a raw food diet, you will definitely experience some challenges and you will need to be cautious. Therefore, in order to succeed while on this diet, we will look at challenges you are likely to face and precautions you need to take while on a raw food diet:

1. A number of people may fall sick when starting on a raw diet, due to a detox reaction as the digestive system gets used to this diet. This is a temporary effect and is exhibited with any diet change.

2. You might experience headaches due to cutting down on caffeine, and an increase in fiber content can cause diarrhea and flatulence in some people. Try to slowly phase in raw foods as you phase out cooked foods, to allow the system to adjust to the change. However, in extreme sickness, the diet might be unsuitable for you.

3. Be mindful on what you consume and the method of preparation. For instance, though nutrients are lost when veggies are cooked, overstoring them in the fridge causes deterioration of nutrients and growth of fungi. Raw food may also lose nutrients when being soaked; frozen, dehydrated, or juiced thus you shouldn't overdo any process.

4. Listen to your body's needs or reaction to this diet, as not everyone is suited to a raw food diet. In case you experience unusual symptoms, talk to your doctor immediately.

5. Learn which foods to avoid, or those to eat in moderation. For example, consuming excess cruciferous veggies and raw kales has been attributed to causing thyroid problems.

6. Avoid this diet in case you are pregnant, if nursing, anemic, if at risk of osteoporosis or a young child. Contact a doctor if you experience any health fragility, immune disorder or other illnesses.

Breakfast Recipes:

Cereal Recipes

Pumpkin Spice Overnight Oats

Servings: 2

Ingredients

½ cup of pumpkin puree (from a sugar pumpkin)

1 ½ cups of almond milk (or other favorite non-diary milk)

¼ teaspoon of nutmeg

¼ teaspoon of ground cloves

½ teaspoon of ginger

½ teaspoon of cinnamon

2 tablespoons of chia seeds

1 cup raw oats

Directions

Stir the chia seeds, oats and spices in a medium bowl. Put the pumpkin puree and almond milk in a bowl and whip them together then whisk into the oat mixture the almond milk mixture. Finally wrap and refrigerate overnight.

Tricks Cereal

Yields 2 cups cereal squares

Ingredients

2 cups of diced fresh organic strawberries

¼ teaspoon of sea salt

1 teaspoon of vanilla extract

6 tablespoons of date paste

1 cup of applesauce

1 ½ cups of packed, moist almond pulp

Directions

Mix the applesauce, date paste, vanilla, salt and the almond pulp in a bowl until well combined then add in the strawberries and mix. Put the mixture onto a dehydrator tray and spread until ¼ inch thick.

Cut the edges and make them into squares then slice into nice small pieces. Dehydrate for about 8-10 hours at 115 degrees until dry, and do the same for the other side. Put in an airtight container and store in the fridge for up to 1-2 weeks.

Oat Meal

Servings: 2

Ingredients

Pure water

2 teaspoons of cinnamon

1 tablespoon of golden flax seed

1 banana

2 apples

Directions

Place the flax seeds in the pure water and let them sit overnight. Peel and cut the apples then split the banana in parts. Take the flax seeds from the water and rinse them out.

Put all the ingredients in a blender then add ¼ cup of water or enough water to blend the mixture. You can add more water if the mixture is too thick.

Raw Granola

Servings: 3

Ingredients

1 teaspoon of cinnamon

1 tablespoon of water

1 tablespoon of flax oil

1/3 cup of maple syrup

1/3 cup of dried, chopped apples

1/3 cup of raisins

1/3 cup of pumpkin seeds

1/3 cup of sunflower seeds

2 tablespoons of ground flaxseed

1 cup soaked and dehydrated buckwheat

Dash of salt

Dash of nutmeg

Directions

Put all the dry ingredients in a large bowl and mix them. Whip together the coconut oil, maple syrup, water, cinnamon, salt and nutmeg. Put in the dry ingredients into the maple mixture and mix them using your hands. To make this mixture sweeter, you can add some drops of stevia.

Dehydrate the mixture for around 10-12 hours at 115 degrees Celsius. You can also dehydrate until the granola is sticky. Refrigerate the mixture until ready to serve.

"Toasted" Apple Cinnamon Cereal

Servings: 5

Ingredients

2 tablespoons of fresh apple juice

¼ cup of blackstrap molasses

¼ cup of hemp oil

¼ teaspoon of Celtic sea salt

¼ teaspoon of ground stevia

¼ teaspoon of ground nutmeg

1 ½ teaspoons of ground cinnamon

½ cup of sunflower seeds

½ cup of unhulled sesame seeds

½ cup of hemp flour

½ cup of ground flaxseed

½ cup of diced raw almonds

1 cup of gluten free oats

½ apple, diced

Directions

Mix the oats, apple, almonds, sesame seeds, ground flaxseed, hemp flour, cinnamon, sunflower seeds, nutmeg, sea salt and stevia until well combined.

Put the molasses, apple juice and the hemp oil into a blender and blend. Mix well the dry ingredients with the wet ingredients and put the mixture in a dehydrator sheet and dehydrate for 24-48 hours at 115 degrees Celsius. The amount of time you choose to dehydrate the cereal will depend on how crunchy you want it to be. Break into pieces and keep in the refrigerator for up to 2 weeks.

Bread And Cake Recipes

Raw Vegan Carrot Cake Cupcakes

Servings: 1

Ingredients

Cupcakes

¾ cup of raisins

1/8 teaspoon of sea salt

Dash of nutmeg

½ teaspoon of ginger

1 teaspoon of cinnamon

2 cups of grated raw carrots; they have to be extremely squeezed through a paper towel to remove as much moisture as possible

1 cup of dates

1 cup of walnuts (not soaked)

Frosting

Water

1 teaspoon of lemon juice

Dash of sea salt

1/3 cup of agave syrup

1 cup of cashews, soaked for about 1 hour

Directions

Put the dates and walnuts in a food processor. Process until they are holding together and flaky. Put in the spices and grated carrots and process until it becomes a smooth dough. Add in the raisins and beat them until they combine with the mixture.

To make the frosting; mix the salt, lemon and rinsed cashews in a food processor. Process the mixture while adding enough water to ensure that the frosting gets the consistency you like. Put the carrot cake dough into ramekins and place in the refrigerator for around an hour. After one hour, remove from the fridge then put frosting on the cupcakes.

Almond Bread

Makes 18 slices

Ingredients

1 cup of flax meal

3 cups of almond flour

2 tablespoons of marjoram

3 tablespoons of Herbs de Provence

1 teaspoon of salt

3 tablespoons of lemon juice

2 apples, cored and roughly chopped

3 medium zucchinis, peeled and roughly chopped

1 cup of sun-dried tomatoes, loosely packed

½ cup of olive oil

Directions

Put into a food processor the olive oil, sun-dried tomatoes, zucchini, apple, lemon juice, salt and dried herbs. Process them until they are mixed well. Now add in the almond flour and process the mixture until you form a batter. Using your hands, add in the flax meal into the batter and mix. Put the mixture into a food processor but in little batches to get a texture that is fluffy and light. Cut the mixture into two and put in a dehydrator tray.

With the use of a cranked palette knife, spread the mixture equally to all of the four sides and corners of the dehydrator tray. If the mixture is very sticky, utilize a wet cranked palette knife. Using a knife, divide the mixture into nine squares. Dehydrate the mixture at 105 degrees for around 2 hours then flip it to be able to dehydrate the other side.

Dehydrate the other side at 105 degrees F for about 8 more hours.

Apple Raisin Bagels

Makes 8 bagels

Ingredients

½ cup of golden raisins

½ cup of coconut flour

1 cup of golden flax meal

¼ teaspoon of salt

1 teaspoon of apple pie spice

½ tablespoon of lemon juice

1 cup of dried jujubes

2 ½ cups of peeled and chopped apple (about two medium apples)

Directions

Put in a blender the lemon juice, salt, apple pie spice and jujubes and blend well. Put the mixture in a bowl and add in the coconut flour, golden raisins and the flaxseed meal. Divide the mixture into 8 portions and make into shapes (bagel).

Put the bagel shapes onto a dehydrator tray for around 24 hours until dehydrated sufficiently. However, the time for dehydration will differ depending on the size of your dehydrator or the humidity.

Raw Lemon Scones with Blackberry Sage "Jam"

Servings: 8

Ingredients

1 cup of almond milk

2 lemons, zest and juice

½ cup of coconut crystals

½ cup of macadamia nuts, ground fine in food processor

1/3 cup of chia seeds

2 ½ cups of raw flaked oats, ground fine to oat flour

Directions for scones

Mix the coconut crystals, ground macadamia nuts and chia seeds in a bowl. Whisk the almond milk, lemon zest and the lemon juice together, and allow it to sit for 5 minutes. Take the wet ingredients and mix into the dry ingredients then leave the mixture for 5 minutes then make into a flat circle then slice into 8 wedges. Put onto a dehydrator and dehydrate for about 45 minutes at 145 degrees. Dehydrate the other side for 7-8 hours at 115 degrees.

Blackberry sage jam Ingredients

1-2 tablespoons maple syrup

1 ½ tablespoons dried sage

1 ½ tablespoons chia seeds

1 pint blackberries

Directions

Process the ingredients in a high-speed blender or food processor until pureed then refrigerate for around 30 minutes for it to set up.

Serve the lemon scones with the jam and enjoy.

Raw banana bread

Servings: 15

Ingredients

¼ cup of sesame seeds

½ cup of chopped pecans

1 cup of raisins

1 pinch of sea salt

1 teaspoon of cinnamon

1 tablespoon of vanilla

½ cup of chia seeds

¼ cup of dates

¼ cup of water

1 2/3 cups of peeled and roughly chopped carrots

5 bananas

Directions

Put in a bowl the raisins, pecans and sesame seeds. Put the sea salt, vanilla, cinnamon, water and the peeled bananas in a blender and blend then add in some dates and carrots and blend until it becomes smooth and creamy then add in the chia seeds and blend until smooth.

Remove the mixture from the blender and mix it with the mixture that you had initially put in a bowl. Mix them well using a spoon. Pour the batter onto a dehydrator tray with teflex sheets. Smooth the batter to ¼ of an inch thick ensuring that you do not make the batter too thin. Dehydrate for 1.5 hours on the highest temperature then dehydrate the other side for some hours at 105 degrees. Keep looking at your bread while on the dehydrator tray to avoid drying the batter so much as you want the bread to be a bit moist.

You can top it with cream cheese or any other toppings that you would like.

Pancake Recipes

Banana Pancakes

Servings: 1

Ingredients

Dash of cinnamon

2 tablespoons of dried coconut flakes

1 banana

Directions

Smash the banana in a bowl using a fork; ensure it is extremely smooth. Mix in some cinnamon and dried coconut flakes to add some flavor.

Make the coconut/ banana dough flat then make small pancakes. Take the small pancakes and leave them out in direct sunlight and after one, hour flip to the other side.

Ensure that they dry completely on the sides.

Raw Blueberry Pancakes

Makes 10 pancakes

Ingredients

2 cups of blueberries, muddled

1 teaspoon of sea salt

Seeds from 2 vanilla beans

1 cup of agave nectar

2 ripe bananas

2 cups of pine nuts

2 cups of pecans, soaked for 4 hours

Directions

Put the pine nuts, bananas, agave nectar, salt, soaked pecans and the remaining soaking liquid and ½ cup of water into a blender. Blend until soft. Fold in the mixed-up blueberries using a spatula.

Using a scoop, put ½ cup scoops onto a dehydrator rack, leaving ½ inch space between the pancakes. Ensure that the pancakes are around ½ inch thick. Dehydrate them for about 8 hours and flip them then dehydrate for another 8 hours. Wrap the pancakes and put them in a refrigerator for up to 3 days.

Banana Pecan Pancakes

Makes 3-4 pancakes

Ingredients

¾ cup of chopped pecans

1 cup of sliced bananas

¼ cup of coconut butter

¼ cup of raw agave nectar

¾ cup of water

½ cup of dried, unsweetened coconut

½ cup of flax seeds

1 ½ cups of ground flax seed

Directions

Mix all the ingredients using your hands in a bowl then make the mixture into pancake size pies. Put on the dehydrator shelf with screen and dehydrate for 30 minutes at 140 degrees, then dehydrate the other side for around 30 minutes at 116 degrees.

Raw Cinnamon Apple Pancakes

Yields 4-6 pancakes

Ingredients

2 tablespoons of ground flax seed

1-2 teaspoons of cinnamon to taste

1 tablespoon of vanilla extract

¼ cup of agave nectar

8 dates, pitted and soaked for at least 30 minutes

¼ soak water from dates

1 cup chopped apples

¼ cup of unsweetened shredded coconut

1 cup of buckwheat groats

Pinch of sea salt

Directions

Put the dates in water and soak them for at least 30 minutes. Put the buckwheat groats in a food processor or blender and grind until finely crumbled. Put them into a different bowl and mix in the shredded coconut.

Take the remaining ingredients including the dates and put them in the food processor and process until you form thick batter. This can be for 20 seconds. Put in the buckwheat coconut mix and mix well. Scoop the mixture onto a dehydrator tray and spread it to the size that you want. It is better if the pancakes are around ½ inch thick. Dehydrate for about 6-8 hours at 115 degrees then flip to the other side and dehydrate for 4-6 hours. Ensure that the pancakes do not dry too much. Store the pancakes in an airtight container and refrigerate for up to 4 days.

Vegan Banana Pancakes

Servings: 1 (about 4-5 pancakes)

Ingredients

¼ cup of almond milk

1 teaspoon of cinnamon

2 tablespoons of flax meal

¼ cup raw buckwheat flour (you make this by grinding the dehydrated buckwheat groats)

1 large banana

Directions

Put all the ingredients in a blender and blend. Put in ¼ cupfuls onto a dehydrator tray. This should give you around 5 pancakes.

Dehydrate the pancakes for around 2 ½ hours at 115 degrees. Then flip the other side, dehydrate also for around 2 ½ hours. You should check the pancakes regularly to avoid over dehydrating them. Finally serve the pancakes with fresh berries.

Blueberry Flax Pancakes

Servings: 1

Ingredients:

¼ cup of coconut; unsweetened and dried

1 cup of blueberries

½ cup of water

¼ cup of agave

3 tablespoons of coconut oil melted

1 cup of flax seeds, not ground

½ cup of flax seeds, ground

Directions

Put all the ingredients in a bowl and mix. Make small pancakes using the mixture then dehydrate the pancakes for about one hour at 145 degrees. Afterwards, flip the pancake and dehydrate at 114 degrees for around 30 minutes.

Raw pancakes

Servings: 6

Ingredients

¼ cup of water

½ teaspoon of sea salt

½ cup of agave nectar

2 tablespoons of coconut oil

3 cups of ground flaxseed meal

Directions

Mix all the ingredients in a large bowl using a spoon. Shape the mixture into pancakes preferably six pancakes. Serve the pancakes with any fresh fruit of your choice for instance blueberries, raspberries or blackberries.

Salad Recipes

Kale Salad

Servings: 2-4

Ingredients

4 tablespoons of lemon juice

Sea salt to taste

2 tablespoons of agave nectar

2-3 tablespoons of olive oil

3 tablespoons of onions, diced

1 avocado, diced

1 tomato, diced

8 leaves each of Russian kale, dino kale and curly kale (shredded)

Directions

Mix all the ingredients in a bowl for about 5 minutes using your hands. Leave the salad for about 2-3 hours to marinate. Finally, garnish the salad with the cherry tomatoes then serve.

Raw Taco Salad

Servings: 2

Ingredients

For salad

2 tablespoons of lemon juice

1/3 bunch of cilantro, chopped

½ red onion, chopped

1 tomato, chopped

2 hearts of romaine (organic)

½ avocado

For the Taco filling

1 teaspoon of chili powder

2 tablespoons of low sodium tamari

½ tablespoon of coriander

1 tablespoon of cumin

2 cups of walnuts

Directions

Place the walnuts in a food processor and process until chunky. Grate the groundnuts into a bowl and add in the coriander, cumin, chili powder and cayenne. Now add in the tamari and mix them again. This is for the taco filling.

Mix the onion, cilantro, lemon juice and the chopped tomatoes (for the salsa). Put the chopped romaine in a bowl, then spoon out the taco filling onto the top. Add in the salsa and top it off with the avocado though the avocado is optional.

Pineapple Passion Fruit Salad

Servings: 4-8

Ingredients

Seeds from two whole passion fruit

2 large green kiwi, peeled

1 pound strawberry

1 large pineapple

Mint leaves for the garnish

Directions

Peel the pineapple using a sharp knife then slice it into four sided cubes and put into a bowl. Peel the kiwi fruit and cut it into ¼-inch slices (horizontally). Take the strawberries, hull them and slice into little pieces, put into a bowl then mix it with the sliced pineapple.

Put the kiwi fruit into the sides of a glass bowl. Add in the strawberries and the pineapple. Cut the passion fruits and put their seeds on top of the salad. Top it off with the fresh mint and serve.

Mint Lemonade Fruit Salad

Yields 5 cups

Ingredients

Pinch of cayenne

1 tablespoon of maple syrup

1/8 teaspoon of fresh lemon zest

2 lemons, juiced

1/3 cup of raw walnuts, chopped

½ avocado, diced

¼ cup of fresh mint leaves, finely chopped

3 cups of fresh organic raspberries

Directions

Put all the ingredients in a bowl and mix. Toss them well then serve immediately or refrigerate to serve later. The raspberries will become softer after tossing the mixture so it is better if the salad is served a few hours after preparing it.

Yum Salad

Servings: 2-4

Ingredients

I handful of nori fronds

Sea salt to taste

3 tablespoons of lemon juice

2 tablespoons of agave nectar

4 tablespoons of sprouted sunflower seeds

3 tablespoons of onions, diced

½ cucumber, diced

1 avocado, diced

1 tomato, diced

1 head romaine lettuce, shredded

Directions

Put all ingredients in a bowl and mix using your hands. The flavors will become stronger after the seaweed breaks up.

Leave the salad for 20 minutes (at room temperature) before serving.

Carrot Salad with Fennel Dressing

Servings: 4

Ingredients for the salad

¼ white onion, finely sliced

½ cup of cherry tomatoes, sliced

¼-1/2 cup of hemp seeds

2 finely sliced Swiss brown mushrooms

1 bunch of fennel tops, chopped

2 finely sliced medium sized fennel bulbs

½ bunch of coriander, chopped

2 medium carrots, spiralised

1 medium zucchini, spiralised

2 cups of mixed leaf salad

Pinch of Himalayan crystal salt

Directions for making the salad

Mix all the ingredients in a bowl.

Fennel Dressing Ingredients

Pinch of Himalayan crystal salt

Water to thin

2 tablespoons of yacon syrup

1 cm piece of ginger

1 clove of garlic

2 tablespoons of chopped fennel

2 tablespoons of fennel tops

4 tablespoons of hemp seed oil

4 tablespoons of apple cider vinegar

1 teaspoon of onion powder

1 teaspoon of garlic powder

1 tablespoon of miso paste

1 tablespoon of tahini

Directions for Fennel Dressing

Mix all the ingredients in a blender, then add some water preferably 2-4 tablespoons and blend the ingredients. Pour the dressing onto the salad bowl and garnish it with a fennel top and additional hemp seeds.

Smoothie Recipes

Green Grapefruit Smoothie

Servings: 1

Ingredients

½ cup of filtered water

1 heaping teaspoon of wheatgrass powder

1 inch of ginger knob

1 large handful of kale

¼ avocado, peeled

½ medium grapefruit, peeled

1 medium banana, frozen

Directions

Put all the ingredients in a blender. Blend them until the desired consistency is reached. This can be for around 45 seconds. Pour into a glass and enjoy.

Coconut-Banana Smoothie

Servings: 1

Ingredients

8 ounces of unsweetened coconut milk

2 cups of kale, stems removed

1 tablespoon of chia seeds, soaked for 5 minutes

1 banana, peeled

1 cup of red grapes

¼ teaspoon of ginger, grated

½ small lime peeled

Directions

Add in the 8 ounces of unsweetened coconut milk, lime followed by chia seeds, kale, banana, red grapes and the ginger to the blender. Blend for 30 minutes until creamy.

If you want the smoothie to be colder, it is better to use frozen bananas or ice cubes.

Chocolate-Acai Green Smoothie

Servings: 1

Ingredients

8 ounces of homemade almond milk

6 medium strawberries

3 cups baby spinach

1 tablespoon raw cacao powder

1 pouch frozen acai puree

1 banana, peeled

Directions

Add the homemade almond milk followed by the strawberries, the frozen acai puree and the banana into the blender then finally add the greens in the blender and blend the mixture for 30 seconds until creamy.

Apricot-Cantaloupe Green Smoothie

Serving: 1

Ingredients

8 ounces of homemade almond nut milk

3 cups of fresh baby spinach

1 medium banana, peeled

1 teaspoon of ground cinnamon

4 apricots, pitted

1 ½ cups of cantaloupe, cubed

Directions

Put all the ingredients into your blender and blend for about 30 seconds or until you achieve a creamy texture.

Chocolate-Cherry Green Smoothie

Servings: 1

Ingredients

8 ounces of unsweetened coconut milk

3 cups of fresh baby spinach

1 tablespoon of cacao powder

1½ cups of beet, peeled

¼ avocado, pitted and peeled (without peel, pit)

1 cup of Bing cherries, pitted

10 strawberries

Directions

Put in the 8 ounces of unsweetened coconut milk to the blender and add in the avocado, Bing cherries and the strawberries. Add to the mixture the baby spinach, beet, and cacao powder. Blend until the mixture is creamy, preferably for 30 seconds.

Kale and Banana Smoothie

Servings: 1

Ingredients

5 leafs of kale

1 teaspoon of super foods

2.5 cups of pure water

1 bag of frozen blueberries

2 tablespoons of hulled hemp seed

2 bananas

Directions

Take all of the ingredients and put in a blender. Put in enough water to ensure that all of the ingredients are covered. Blend the ingredients extremely well and you can add water if you would like a smoothie that is a bit thinner.

Almond Vanilla Smoothie

Yields 1 quart

Ingredients

1 tiny pinch of salt (optional)

½ cup of young coconut meat

1 banana

3 tablespoons of honey

2 cups of water

1 teaspoon of vanilla

½ cup of almonds

Directions

For the almond milk: Put all the almonds with the water in a blender and blend. Take a nylon nut milk bag and strain the almond milk then put aside the pulp and return the almond milk back into the blender. Put in the other ingredients and blend well.

Porridge And Pudding Recipes

Coconut Chia Seed Pudding

Servings: 1

Ingredients

1 teaspoon of vanilla

½ tablespoon of cinnamon

1 teaspoon of coconut nectar

1 cup of almond milk

3 tablespoons of chia seeds

Toppings

1 plum

1 teaspoon of walnuts, cranberries, coconut and pepitas

1 pear

Directions

Mix all the ingredients using a fork in a bowl. Leave the mixture for about 20 minutes and stir it after every 5 minutes. You can add the toppings once the chia seeds have soaked up all the liquid.

Chia Seed Breakfast Pudding

Servings: 2

Ingredients

Granola for the topping if desired

1/3 cup of chia seeds

3 oranges

3 dates, softened with pits removed

1 cup of water

¼ cup of almonds, soaked overnight, drained and rinsed

Directions

Put the almonds in a blender and blend then strain the nut milk. Put back the almonds in the blender and blend together with the dates until smooth and creamy. Now add in the zest from one of the oranges into the almond dates mixture.

Partition the inside parts of 1 orange then juice out the other two oranges. Add in the orange juice into the zest and almond mixture and mix. Add in the chia seeds and let the mixture sit for around 20 minutes. Add in the orange sections that you had partitioned.

Raw chocolate pudding

Servings: 2

Ingredients

Cocoa to taste

Cinnamon to taste

3 tablespoons of chia seed, gelled with water

¼ cup of raisins

2 tablespoons of agave

1 teaspoon of vanilla extract

2 tablespoons of almond butter

2 bananas

Directions

Put the chia seeds in a bowl, add in water, ¼ cup or more until they are covered and leave them to gel. Put the other ingredients in a food processor and process until soft. After the chia seeds are gelled, add them to the food processor and process. Serve the mix in bowls and garnish with goji berries or any other fruit, and coconut flakes

Morning Burst Porridge

Serving: 1

Ingredients

1 ripe banana, chopped

2 tablespoons of walnuts, chopped

½ teaspoon of vanilla extract

2 tablespoons of chia seeds

1 tablespoon of carob powder

1/3 cup of raw rolled oats

1 cup of almond nut milk

Toppings: raisins, buckwheat (soaked and dehydrated) and shredded coconut (optional

Dash of salt

Directions

Mix all the dry ingredients in a bowl. Put in the other ingredients and mix them well. Put the mixture in the fridge for about 1 hour or if even overnight. You can garnish with whatever you want, serve and enjoy!

Other Breakfast Recipes

Raw muesli, with fresh mango and raw almond nut cream

Servings: 1

Ingredients

Raw nut milk to taste

1 tablespoon of fresh raw grated coconut (optional)

Fresh fruit (banana, berries or mango)

2 tablespoons of coconut oil (optional)

About 10 dates, soaked and pitted

¾ cups of raw nuts

Directions

Put the dates, coconut oil and the nuts in a food processor and process them; the nuts should be finely grounded. Place the mixture in a bowl and add in grated coconut and fresh fruit. Top it up with nut milk.

Almond Cherry Macaroons

Yields 2 dozen

Ingredients

¼ cup of coconut oil

½ cup of agave

½ cup of dried cherries, chopped

½ cup of almonds, processed into a coarse meal

2 cups of dried coconut (unsweetened)

Directions

Put the almonds in a food processor and mix until they have a coarse meal texture. Put in the dried cherries, coconut, coconut oil, agave and the almond extract. Process until the mixture holds together.

Take a tablespoon, scoop the mixture and make into many balls. Put them on a dehydrator and dehydrate for preferably 8-10 hours.

Sun-dried Tomato Olive Crackers

Makes one sheet

Ingredients

1 teaspoon of oregano

½ cup of olives, sliced

1/3 cup of softened and chopped sun-dried tomatoes

¼ cup of water

½ cup of ground flax

2 cups of walnuts; soaked overnight, drained and rinsed

Himalayan salt and pepper to taste

Pinch thyme

Directions

Put the walnuts in a food processor and process until they are finely ground. Add in the ground flax and process again until well mixed. Put in the olives and sun-dried tomatoes and process again.

Mix in the thyme, salt, pepper and the oregano. Spread the mixture on a dehydrator sheet (non-stick) and compress into 1/4-1/8 inch thick. Dehydrate the mixture for about one hour at 140 degrees, then turn and dehydrate the other side at 115 degrees until extremely dry.

Almond Pulp Crackers

Yields 30 crackers

Ingredients

¼ cup of water (and more as needed)

2 tablespoons of ground flax meal

1/3 - ½ teaspoons of salt

½ cup of buckwheat flour

1 cup of almond pulp (well strained)

Directions

Put all the ingredients in a blender and blend until smooth. Add in some water then continue adding until you get the correct dough texture. The dough should not be very dry to spread on a dehydrator tray and it should be firm to retain its shape.

Partition the dough into two halves and spread it onto a dehydrator tray until it is around ¼ inch thick. Divide the dough into squares. Dehydrate for about 5-6 hours at 115 degrees then flip the dough and dehydrate at the same temperature for around 5-6 hours until it is completely dry. Break into crackers, serve and enjoy!

Cucumber Sandwich

Servings: 2

Ingredients

Few cilantro leaves

Salt and cayenne pepper

Squeeze of lime

1 small tomato, cubed

1 avocado, cubed

1 cucumber

Directions

Slice the cucumber lengthwise and horizontally. You should have 4 lengthy "boats". Using a spoon, take out the soft inner part of the cucumber. Mix the rest of the ingredients in a bowl gently. Take the other ingredients and mix them gently in a bowl.

Fill up the soft inner part of the cucumber with the mixture that was in the bowl. Put the other empty half on top of the cucumber then enjoy.

Lunch Recipes:

Salad Recipes

Avocado-Hemp Salad

Servings: 2

Ingredients

1 cubed, small jicama

1 nori sheet, little pieces

1 teaspoon of hemp seeds

1 avocado

2-3 cups of shredded organic lettuce

Cherry tomatoes, sea salt, lime juice and spices (optional)

Directions

Put the lettuce in a bowl then add in the avocado and mash it then add in the nori and the cubed jicama garnish with the hemp seeds. Juice the lime and add in some spices for a better flavor.

Chili Marinated Cucumber Salad

Servings: 1

Ingredients

½ teaspoon of black pepper

1 teaspoon of chili flakes

3 tablespoons of maple syrup

2 tablespoons of fruity flavored EVOO

1/3 cup of apple cider vinegar

¼ cup of sliced sweet onion

2 cups cucumbers (seedless or lighter seeds), paper-thinly sliced

1 teaspoon of hemp seeds (optional)

Pinch of sea salt

Spritz of lemon juice

Directions

Wash the cucumbers, and slice them thinly then put them in a bowl. Mix in some sliced onion, add in some spritz of the lemon juice, and mix.

In another bowl, put in all the spices, maple syrup, the EVOO, and the apple cider vinegar then mix well. Transfer the cucumbers in a large bowl then add in the liquid with spices ensuring that the liquid covers each cucumber. Put the salad in the fridge for about 2-3 hours then serve with arugula or serve alone.

Cheezy broccoli

Servings: 2

Ingredients

1 peeled and minced clove of garlic

1 teaspoon of ashwaganda extract powder

3 teaspoons of nutritional yeast such as Engevita

120ml | ½ cup water for the recipe and additional soaking water

80g | 3/4 cup of raw cashew nuts

1 teaspoon of apple cider vinegar

4 teaspoons of olive oil

200g | 3 cups of broccoli

Directions

Put the nuts in water and soak them overnight then rinse them. Slice the broccoli into little florets and combine it with the apple cider vinegar and olive oil then set it aside for some time.

Put all the other ingredients into a blender and blend them until smooth. Put the mixture into a shallow dish, and cover using a dark fabric. Put the dish in a dark warm cabinet for about 8 hours or if you want, leave it overnight. Once the mixture tastes cheesy, add in the broccoli, mix and then serve and enjoy!

Courgetti with basil pesto

Servings: 4

Ingredients

4 large julienned courgettes

½ fresh finely chopped chili (optional)

Salt and black pepper

2 tablespoons of fresh lemon juice

9 tablespoons of olive oil

1 large garlic clove

50g of fresh basil

12 cashew nuts, soaked for 6 hours

Directions

Drain the soaked cashew nuts, and rinse them then process the cashew nuts with the lemon juice, olive oil, garlic and the basil in a food processor. You can then add chili, pepper, and salt then mix. Now fold the pesto into the julienned courgettes, serve, and enjoy.

Raw salad

Servings: 1

Ingredients

1 avocado

1 medium tomato

1-2 carrots

Directions

Slice the tomato and carrot into small pieces and put in a bowl. Chop the avocado into two halves, remove the pit, and slice it into other two halves then into smaller pieces. Add the avocado into the bowl then mix all the three ingredients. Sprinkle some salt and pepper and eat right away.

Mexican Salad

Servings: 4

Ingredients

1 tablespoon of dried coriander

¼ red onion

1 teaspoon of cumin

40g of pumpkin seeds

10g of fresh coriander

40g of celery

½ pineapple

2 limes

2 avocados

Directions

Cut the avocado, remove the pit, peel and mash roughly. Remove the core from the pineapple and slice it into cubes. Chop the onion and the celery into fine pieces then slice the coriander roughly. Place all of these ingredients in a bowl, and juice one lime onto the ingredients.

Slice the leftovers of the lime into quarters and put them into the middle of the bowl. Refrigerate in a sealed container for about two days.

Cucumber Salad

Servings: 6

Ingredients

6 cucumbers, chopped

6 tomatoes, diced

2 teaspoons celery seeds

2 tablespoons dill

1 cup parsley, chopped

2 tablespoons lemon juice

4 tablespoons olive oil

2 radishes, finely sliced

2 carrots, grated

½ cup scallions, chopped

Salt and pepper to taste

Directions

Mix the tomatoes, cucumbers, scallions, radishes and olive oil in a bowl then blend the rest of the ingredients for the dressing. Pour the dressing over the salad and enjoy.

Beetroot with walnut crumble and tahini sauce

Servings: 2

Ingredients

For the beetroots

2 tablespoons of lemon juice

2 tablespoons of olive oil

2 raw, peeled and thinly sliced golden beetroots

2 raw, peeled and thinly sliced red beetroots

Sea salt to taste

For the crumble

1 garlic clove (crushed)

A pinch of ground chipotle

1 teaspoon of ground cumin

12g of nutritional yeast flakes

100g of raw, soaked, and dried walnuts

2-3 tablespoons of water

Sea salt to taste

For the dressing

½ teaspoon of ground cumin

2 tablespoons of lemon juice

2 tablespoons of water

2 tablespoons of tahini

Sea salt to taste

To assemble

A handful of baby spinach leaves

1 sliced shallot

1 sliced avocado

Directions

Put the golden beetroot in a bowl and place the red beetroot in another bowl. Sprinkle 1 tablespoon of lemon juice and 1 tablespoon of oil on top of each bowl together with some salt. Toss and leave for some time.

For the crumble

Process all the ingredients apart from water in a blender then add 1 tablespoon of water at a time until the mixture starts to form clumps then leave it once it becomes clumpy.

For the tahini dressing

Mix all of the ingredients until they are smooth.

To assemble

Place the beetroot slices in circle in two plates while interchanging between the golden and red discs. Garnish with baby spinach leaves, shallot slices and the avocado. Sprinkle the tahini dressing and top with the crumble.

Raw Soup Recipes

Mango Ginger Soup

Servings: 2

Ingredients

½ teaspoon of minced ginger

Lime juice from one lime

1-2 small minced chili peppers to add flavor

½ cup of cold water

½ chopped onion

1 large peeled and destoned mango

Directions

Put all the ingredients into a blender and blend until very creamy and smooth. Add water according to how thick you want the soup to be. Put the soup in a fridge then serve after some minutes.

Avocado Carrot Soup

Servings: 2

Ingredients

1 tablespoon of coconut sugar (optional)

¼ lemon

1 teaspoon of finely chopped ginger

¼ cup of sesame milk

2 medium carrots

Pure Water

Pinch of cayenne pepper

1 avocado

Directions

Place all of the ingredients in a blender and blend. Add in some water if the mixture is very thick and keep adding water until you get the consistency that you want.

If you want your soup to become warm, you can add some warm water into the blender preferably 150 F or 50 C and ensure that the water is not too warm as it is better when the enzymes stay alive. Furthermore, the avocado becomes bitter when hot.

Cucumber soup

Servings: 2

Ingredients

Broccoli sprouts

5g of Sea greens

10ml hemp seed oil

10ml of Udo's Choice oil

¼ small red onion

1 clove of garlic

1 celery stalk

1 small tomato

½ red pepper

½ avocado

½ cucumber

70g of shelled hempseeds

400ml of water not quite boiled from a kettle

Directions

Peel the avocado and put all the ingredients into a blender. Blend until smooth and pour into two bowls. Top with some extra oil and more sea greens before serving.

Raw Green Pea Soup

Servings: 2

Ingredients

1 small onion

1 ½ cups of almond milk

1 avocado

2 cups of peas

1 teaspoon of salt or to taste

½ teaspoon of pepper or to taste

Directions

Put aside ½ cup of peas and blend the avocado, almond milk, salt, pepper, and the remaining peas. Blend until the mixture is smooth. Put in some pepper and salt to add flavor to the soup. Pour soup into bowls and garnish with minced onion and the peas that you had set aside.

Butternut Squash soup

Servings: 6

Ingredients

1 large butternut squash, peeled

10 apples, cored

¼ cup tarragon, dried

1 bunch parsley

1 ½ cups pumpkin seeds

3 cups almond milk

1 red onion, peeled

1 lemon, peeled

2 oranges, peeled

Directions

Combine all the ingredients in a food processor and puree then pour into bowls and enjoy.

Celery Soup

Servings: 2

Ingredients

1 bunch celery, chopped

½ cup lemon juice

¼ cup olive oil

4 cups water

Salt and pepper to taste

1 tablespoon honey

1 tomato sliced

1 avocado

Directions

Blend all the ingredients then serve. Garnish with parsley sprig.

Vegetable Soup

Servings: 2

Ingredients

1 date, pitted

1 handful sun dried tomatoes

¼ teaspoon red pepper flakes

1 garlic clove, minced

1 tablespoon apple cider vinegar

2 cups filtered water

1/24 cup chopped fresh basil

4 scallions, sliced

2 cups cherry tomatoes, quartered

1 zucchini, diced

2 bell peppers, diced

2 cups fresh corn kernels

Sea salt to taste

1 tablespoon miso

2 tablespoons nutritional yeast

Directions

Combine the scallions, basil, tomatoes, zucchini, peppers, and corn in a bowl. Remove a third of this mixture and put in a blender with the other remaining ingredients. Blend until smooth then add to the bowl with the veggies. Let it sit for several hours in the fridge to allow the flavors to mix then serve.

Corn Chowder

Servings: 2

Ingredients

½ teaspoon of cumin

½ teaspoon of chili pepper

Dash of soy sauce

Dash of sesame oil

1 handful, soaked, sun dried tomatoes

1 crushed clove of garlic

2 cups of fresh corn

2 ½ cups of almond milk

Toppings

Finely chopped parsley

Thinly sliced Zucchini

Yellow squash, thinly sliced

Red pepper, thinly sliced

Mushrooms, sliced

Sweet onion, sliced

Directions

Place the ingredients in a blender, and blend them then add the toppings and blend again. You can add some seasonings or ½ jalapeño diced if you want the mixture to be spicier.

SMOOTHIE RECIPES

Pear, date, and nut smoothie

Servings: 1

Ingredients

2 tablespoons of Hemp protein powder

1 pear

2 organic Medjool dates

Dash of cinnamon

Dash of flaxseed oil

½ cucumber

½ zucchini

¼ avocado

1 tablespoon of nut butter

2 handfuls of baby spinach

500mls of filtered water

Stevia to taste (optional)

Directions

Put all the ingredients in a blender and blend until you achieve the consistency you like.

Strawberry Beet Detox Smoothie

Servings: 1

Ingredients

8 ounces of coconut water

¼ cup of dry old-fashioned oats

10 fresh or frozen medium strawberries

1 stalk of celery

¼ peeled and pitted avocado

½ cup of chopped beets

Directions

Pour the coconut water put into a blender and add in the strawberries and avocado. Blend for some seconds then add the oats, celery and the beets. Blend again for 30 seconds on high speed until it becomes creamy. Serve and enjoy!

Raw Food Green Smoothie

Yields 4 cups

Ingredients

¼ cup of lightly packed mint leaves

¼ cup of lightly packed cilantro

2 cups of sliced banana

1 ½ cups of tightly packed kales

2 cups of freshly squeezed orange juice

¼ cup of lightly packed parsley

Directions

Place all the ingredients in a blender, and blend for about 10-20 seconds. Ensure that the greens have been blended completely. You can serve right away or refrigerate and serve later.

Apple Pie Green Smoothie

Servings: 1

Ingredients

¼ chopped and frozen avocado

1 chopped and frozen apple,

2 cups spinach

½ English cucumber

Pinch of ground nutmeg

¼ teaspoon of vanilla extract

½ teaspoon of ground cinnamon

1 tablespoon of walnuts

½ cup of unsweetened unpasteurized apple juice

½ cup water

4-6 ice cubes

Directions

Put all the ingredients in a blender, and blend for about 30 seconds or until the mixture is creamy and smooth. Serve and enjoy!

Spinach Smoothie

Servings: 2-4

Ingredients

1 pound of fresh spinach

Small chunk of fresh ginger

2 bananas

4 stalks of celery

2 oranges

Purified water

Directions

Put the ingredients in a blender and blend well until smooth then serve.

Raw Meat Recipes

Steak Tartare

Servings: 8

Ingredients

½ teaspoon of Dijon mustard

¼ cup of chopped parsley

1 tablespoon of red wine vinegar

Dash of hot sauce

Worcestershire sauce, to add flavor

6 anchovy filets, cut in small pieces

Black pepper, to taste

Sea salt, to taste

2 tablespoons of extra virgin olive oil

2 egg yolks, preferably from organic, pasture-raised eggs

1 chopped small onion

2 tablespoons of capers

2 pounds of prime grass-fed sirloin

Directions

Cut the meat finely using a sharp knife. Combine all the ingredients cautiously to retain fluffiness. Form the mixture into a big loaf then top with more capers, onions, and anchovy strips. Serve with any type of cracker.

Salmon Ceviche with Tomato & Avocado

Servings: 6

Ingredients

Fish and citrus juice

¾ to 1 cup of lemon juice

1 ½ to 2 pounds of rinsed, cut into 1-inch cubes, and skinned wild salmon fillets

Vegetables and seasonings

Wheat-free tamari soy sauce, to taste

½ teaspoon of finely ground, unrefined sea salt

½ teaspoon of ground black pepper

¼ cup of minced fresh dill weed

1 ½ teaspoons of dry mustard or 3 large or 4 medium-size red, peeled, seeded, and diced tomatoes

Garnish

Additional lemon juice

2 medium-large halved, pitted, peeled and sliced avocados

Directions

Put the salmon in a bowl, mix in some lemon juice and toss to ensure that the salmon is completely coated with the lemon juice. Cover with a lid and put in a refrigerator for about 6-12 hours. Turn the fish two times using a spoon to ensure that fish is entirely marinated. If the fish is ready, it will appear translucent.

Dry the fish and pat dry to ensure it is dry. Put the seasonings and the vegetables in a glass bowl. Add in the salmon, cover with lid, and then put in the refrigerator for about 2-4 hours. Add the tamari soy sauce and the sea salt then cut the avocado into slices and put into the same bowl. Toss with some lemon juice and garnish with salad greens. Cover with a lid the left overs and refrigerate. Ensure that the leftovers are used within 48 hours.

Don ceviche

Servings: 4

Ingredients

For the tiger's milk

Juice of 8 limes

4 roughly chopped coriander sprigs

1 halved small garlic cloves

½ cm halved fresh ginger

2 small medium-strength deseeded chilies

½ teaspoon of salt

For the ceviche

1 cooked and cut into small cubes, sweet potato (optional)

1 handful of finely chopped coriander leaves

Salt

600g skinned, trimmed and cut into 3x2cm strips sea bass fillet

1 large red onion, very thinly sliced

Directions

For the tiger's milk, place the lime juice, coriander, garlic, and the ginger into a large bowl, mix these ingredients, and then set aside.

Wash the sliced onion and let it sit in iced water for it to soak for about 5 minutes. Drain the water and place the sliced onion onto a towel then put in the fridge until you want to use it.

Place in a bowl the strip of fish, put in some salt and mix smoothly using a spoon. Set aside the fish for about two minutes and add in the tiger's milk. Mix softly using a spoon then set it aside for around 2 minutes. Add in the cubed sweet potato, coriander and the onions. Mix gently and taste to ensure that it tastes the way you want. Distribute between four bowls and eat right away.

Vegan Raw heart of palm and Jicama Ceviche

Servings: 2

Ingredients

½ large avocado

¼ cup of finely chopped red onion

¼ jalapeño pepper

Juice from 1-2 limes

4 hearts of palm, canned, and finely chopped

¼ cup fresh cilantro, finely chopped

1 finely chopped tomato

1 cup of peeled and cubed jicama

Sea salt & pepper to taste

Directions

Combine the red onion, tomato, cilantro, lime juice, jalapeno pepper and the hearts of palm in a bowl. Leave the mixture for about 10-20 minutes in the fridge to enable it to absorb all the flavors then season with some sea salt. Remove the pit from the avocado, peel it and then cut the avocado into cubes and put into the mixture then mix well and garnish with lettuce leaves or tostadas.

Steak Tartare with Pickled Jalapeños

Servings: 2

Ingredients

4 ounces of hangar steak

Filtered water

2 teaspoons of shallots

4 teaspoons of parmagano regiano

4 teaspoons of pickled jalapeño

Salt, pepper, and lemon as needed

¼ lemon squeezed

A dash of soy sauce

½ teaspoon of Tabasco sauce

½ teaspoon of dashi

1 teaspoon of olive oil

Directions

Wash the hangar steak with some filtered water and pat dry with paper towel. Cover tightly and put in the fridge for around 20-30 minutes or until the meat is cool enough such that it is easy to cut.

Mix the 4 teaspoons of the grated parmagano regiano, 4 teaspoons of the diced pickled jalapeno, and 2 teaspoons of the shallots in a bowl. Add in the olive oil, dashi, tabasco sauce, soy sauce, and lemon then mix. You can add more salt, pepper, and lemon depending on what you want. Now cut the steak with a sharp knife and put into a bowl then add in the parmagano regiano mixture and top with ½ teaspoon of sesame seeds and some more grated parmagano.

Burritos and Wraps

Mushroom Taco Lettuce Wraps

Servings: 4-6

Ingredients

For the marinated mushrooms

1 teaspoon of apple cider vinegar

2 tablespoons of maple syrup

3 tablespoons of low-sodium soy sauce

3 cups of roughly chopped mushrooms

Optional: 1 teaspoon of cold pressed olive oil

Ensure that you soak your walnuts for about 3 hours before making wraps and marinate the mushrooms.

Directions

Place the mushrooms into a container that can be sealed. Mix all the ingredients for marinating the mushrooms, then pour on top of the mushrooms. Close the container and shake to ensure that the mushrooms are coated with the marinated liquid. Leave for about 2-3 hours in the refrigerator and shake frequently to ensure that the mushrooms are completely coated.

For the walnut filling

1 handful of fresh parsley

1 teaspoon of chipotle powder

1 teaspoon of smoked paprika

1 teaspoon of coriander

1 teaspoon of cumin

Marinated mushrooms from above recipe

2 cups soaked for 2-3 hours, rinsed and drained walnuts

Optional: 1 cup of cooked quinoa

Himalayan salt and pepper to add flavor

Directions

Put the walnuts in a food processor and process until chunky. Make sure that you do not over process. Put in the parsley, mushrooms, and process until mixed well. Mix in the salt, pepper, quinoa and the other spices.

Assembly

1 avocado

1 cup of quartered cherry tomatoes

1 head of butter lettuce

Walnut mixture

Himalayan salt and pepper

Directions for the assembly

Put the walnut mixture in a lettuce leaf. Garnish with cherry tomatoes and avocado. Top with a grind of pepper and salt.

Mushroom Burritos

Yields 5 burritos

Ingredients

For the burrito Wraps

Mixed veggies of your choice

5 de-stemmed Collard greens

For the dipping Sauce

2 Medjool dates

¼ - ½ cup of water

2-4 tablespoons nutritional yeast

⅔ cup of sun dried tomatoes

¼ red onion

1-2 medium carrots

1 red bell pepper

For the Spicy mushroom Filling

1 handful of raisins

Chopped green onion

1-2 garlic cloves

1-2 teaspoons of raw coconut aminos

Few de-stemmed thyme springs

¼ lemon

3.2 ounces mushrooms

Dash of red chili flakes

Directions

For the spicy mushroom, slice the mushrooms and marinate them using the chili flakes, raisins, green onion, and the garlic cloves. Stir frequently to ensure that the mushrooms are completely marinated.

Blend the sauce ingredients then you can slice some vegetables for example carrots, onions, or cabbage for the burrito wraps.

For the burritos, place a collard green flat, and line it up with the veggies that you have sliced. Garnish the burritos with the spicy mushroom mix then roll it up. Dip the burrito in the sauce, serve, and enjoy!

Lettuce Wraps

Servings: 4

Ingredients

For the salad

Sea salt to taste

4 tablespoons lime juice, freshly squeezed

4 tablespoons mirin

4 tablespoons soy sauce

15g fresh ginger, thinly julienned

1 small piece of daikon radish, thinly julienned

1 large carrot, thinly julienned

1 green papaya, peeled, deseeded and thinly julienned

1 small chili, deseeded and finely chopped

2 tablespoons agave nectar

1 tablespoon sesame oil

For the wraps

1 handful sunflower sprouts

1 handful mint

1 handful basil

80g fresh coconut, sliced

1 head of lettuce

Sea salt to taste

1 tablespoon nut oil

50g raw almonds, chopped

Directions

Whisk together the lime juice, mirin, soy sauce, chopped chilli, agave and sesame oil then add the julienned vegetables into the bowl, sprinkle with some salt then toss to mix. Allow the salad to sit for around 30 minute then drain before using.

Mix the almonds with the oil then add salt to taste.

Separate lettuce leaves then wash and dry them. In the middle of each leaf, place a little salad, avocado, sprouts, and herbs then sprinkle with almonds and wrap.

Nori Rolls

Servings: 4-6

Ingredients

For the rice

1 tablespoon of raw soy sauce

1-2 pinches of Celtic sea salt

2 tablespoons of lemon juice

1 ½ tablespoons of agave nectar

1 tablespoon of hemp seed oil

3 tablespoons of pine nuts

3 tablespoons of Mac nuts

1 ¾ cups of peeled fresh parsnips

For the Extras

½ cup of sprouts e.g. alfalfa sprouts

1 avocado julienned

Nori

Grated wasabi

Marinated Veggies for Sushi

1 yellow zucchini (all the veggies should be sliced into ¼ inch-by-3-inch matchsticks)

1 cucumber

1 scallion, white and pale-green parts

1 stalk celery, strings removed

1 red bell pepper

1 medium carrot, peeled

Marinate everything for about 1-2 hours in:

2 tablespoons of lemon juice

1 tablespoon of raw soy sauce

1 tablespoon of black sesame seeds

3 tablespoons of sesame oil

Refrigerate all of the ingredients until ready to use them

Directions

Process all of the ingredients for the rice in a food processor until the mixture becomes rice-like then set it aside. Take a piece of the nori and then put it on a surface. Put onto a quarter of the nori piece 2-3 tablespoons of the rice mixture. Create a small indent and add in 1-2 tablespoons of the marinated veggies.

Garnish with some bits of the avocado. Add in the 2 pinches of sprouts then roll up the sushi with your fingers or sushi mat and ensure that you make the roll tighter every time when roll it. Leave the roll for about 5 minutes before you cut it. Take a knife and slice the nori into 5-6 equivalent parts. Put on a plate 5 nori rolls then top with edible flowers, sesame seeds and garlic chives. Serve the nori rolls with the raw soy sauce and grated wasabi.

Raw Pasta Recipes

Mermaid Pasta with Veggies

Servings: 1

Ingredients

12 ounces kelp noodles

1 carrot, 1 small zucchini, 1 red bell pepper (sliced into fine strips)

3 scallions, thickly sliced transversely

Handful of fresh baby Bok Choy

2 medium sized pieces of wakame

6 fresh shiitake mushrooms soaked in warm water for ten minutes

For the Dressing

3 cloves of minced garlic

1 tablespoon of raw honey

1 tablespoon of fresh lime juice

3 tablespoons of tamari

2 Tablespoons of cold-pressed sesame oil

Fresh black pepper to taste

Directions

Place the noodles in a colander, rinse in warm water, then drain the water. After soaking the mushrooms and the wakame in warm water for ten minutes until soft, then slice them into thin slices then chop the seaweed and combine it with, wakame, mushrooms, bell pepper, zucchini, carrot, onions, and the Bok Choy.

Mix the dressing ingredients in a bowl then sprinkle this on top of the veggies. It is advisable to marinate the veggies for some hours before serving

Raw Pasta with Nut Balls

Servings: 2-4

Ingredients

For the noodles

1 zucchini

1 bell pepper

1 carrot

For the sauce

½ cup mushrooms

Pinch of salt & pepper

Olive oil

2 tablespoons of sun-dried tomatoes

1 clove garlic

Basil, oregano, other spices

1 tomato

For the nut balls

Olive oil (or water)

2 cloves garlic

Cumin, coriander, turmeric, cayenne, etc. and other spices you may like

¼ cup walnuts

¼ cup almonds

Pinch of salt & pepper

Directions

For the noodles

Cut all the ingredients for the noodles into very thin slices using a sharp knife. Drizzle some salt and some olive oil and let them sit for some time.

For the nut balls

Put the garlic, walnuts, and almonds into a food processor and process until the mixture is in an extremely rough flour size. Mix in the spices and salt then add some olive oil and process until the mix is powdery but sticks together when shaping it. Make nut balls with the mixture and put in the refrigerator for about 1hour. You can also dehydrate the nut balls for around 2-4 hours

For the sauce

Process the sundried tomatoes, salt, garlic, spices, mushrooms and the tomato in a food processor until the mixture becomes a thick sauce. Mix in the olive oil until it gets the consistency you like.

Assembly

Pour over the sauce onto the noodles and combine them well until the noodles are coated with the sauce. Serve the pasta and sauce with the nut balls.

Raw Zucchini Pasta with Curry Cream Sauce

Servings: 1

Ingredients

For the raw zucchini pasta

1 medium zucchini

Sea salt to taste

Extra virgin oil for flavor

A spiral slicer

For the sauce

Freshly chopped mint

Mild curry to taste

A splash of coconut milk to thin

½ to 1 cup of Cashew cream sauce

For the cashew cream sauce

Fresh filtered water

1 cup of organic raw cashews

For the plate

Fresh cilantro

Slices of mango

Sweet yellow tomatoes

Fresh baby salad greens

Directions

Peel the zucchini, then cut the both ends equally, making a straight diagonal edge at the top and bottom of the zucchini. Cut the zucchini in half then empty the zucchini strands into a bowl. Sprinkle a bit of extra virgin oil onto the zucchini pasta and drizzle in some sea salt to add flavor then toss the zucchini strands and set them aside.

To make the sauce, soak the cashews in a bowl for two hours ensuring that you cover the bowl with a clean towel. After the two hours, drain and the sauce is ready. Then take spoonful or two of coconut milk and use this to start thinning the cashew crème sauce. Spice up the sauce with fresh herbs and curry to add flavor. Start putting a small bit of the sauce onto the zucchini and toss. This will depend on the amount of sauce you want on the zucchini but do not completely soak the pasta with the sauce.

Put onto a plate the sweet yellow tomatoes and the salad greens. Put in at the center a serving of the zucchini pasta. Top with slices of mango, and drizzle the top with some fresh cilantro then serve.

OTHER LUNCH RECIPES

Raw Pad Thai

Servings: 4

Ingredients

2 zucchini, ends trimmed

1 thinly sliced head red cabbage

2 carrots

2 oranges, juiced

1 thinly sliced red bell pepper

¾ cup of raw almond butter

1 minced clove of garlic

2 tablespoons of raw honey

½ cup of bean sprouts

1 tablespoon of minced fresh ginger root

1 tablespoon of unpasteurized miso

¼ teaspoon of cayenne powder

1 tablespoon of raw soy sauce

Directions

44444444444

Cut the zucchini horizontally using a peeler to make long slender noodles then put the zucchini on plates. Cut the carrots the same way as the zucchini then mix the carrots with the cabbage, bean sprouts and the red bell pepper.

Take another bowl and whisk together the orange juice, cayenne powder, garlic, miso, honey, ginger, raw soy sauce, and the almond butter. Pour half the sauce over the cabbage mix and toss to ensure that the cabbage mixture is coated with the sauce. Top the zucchini noodles on the plates with the cabbage mix then pour the remaining sauce on each of the plates

Cauliflower tabbouleh

Servings: 2

Ingredients

For the tabbouleh

1 tablespoon of pomegranate seeds, nuts

1 large handful of finely chopped mint leaves,

4 large handfuls of finely chopped parsley

½ medium deseeded and diced cucumber

4 large tomatoes, seeds removed and diced

1 medium red onion

2 teaspoons of ghee

1 medium head of finely grated cauliflower (about 400g)

For the dressing

Salt and black pepper

½ teaspoon of ground cumin

¼ teaspoon of ground cinnamon

1 teaspoon of raw honey

1 garlic clove, crushed

6 tablespoons of extra virgin olive oil

1½ tablespoons of apple cider vinegar

Directions

Put the cauliflower in a bowl and add in the other ingredients for the tabbouleh but not the pomegranate seeds. Combine all the ingredients for the dressing and pour onto the tabbouleh then season with salt and pepper. Sprinkle the pomegranate seeds that you had set aside then serve.

Raw Mashed "Potatoes"

Servings: 1

Ingredient

1 head cauliflower, broken into florets

¼ cup of olive oil to taste

2 cloves of peeled and minced garlic

¼ cup of cashews

Black pepper to taste

Sea salt to taste

Directions

Put the cashews into a food processor and process until the cashews are fine. Mix in the garlic and the cauliflower and process until the mixture is fine. Put in olive oil until the mix becomes fluffy. Remove the mixture from the food processor and drizzle some black pepper. Serve this dish with gravy.

Dinner Recipes:

Salad Recipes

Sea Vegetable Salad

Servings: 2

Ingredients

For salad

2 tablespoons black sesame seeds

2 tablespoons white sesame seeds

Bunch watercress, chopped

1 green onion, sliced

1 white radish, julienned

3 beets, julienned

1 tablespoon wakame, soaked and drained

3 tablespoons arame, soaked and drained

For the sour cherry marinade

2 drops stevia

¼ cup Apple Cider Vinegar

3 tablespoons raw agave syrup

½ cup dehydrated sour cherries or inca berries

For miso dressing

Few drops of toasted sesame oil

3 tablespoon dark raw agave

¼ cup sesame oil

1 clove garlic

¼ cup chopped ginger

1 lemon juice

¼ cup apple cider vinegar

½ cup miso shiro

Directions

1. Into a bowl, mix together the apple cider vinegar, raw agave syrup, cherries or berries and sweeten with the stevia.

2. Soak the mixture for about 1 hour, and then drain and set it aside.

3. Prepare the ingredients for miso dressing, mix together into a blender and then set aside once ready.

4. To make the salad, mix together the salad ingredients into a bowl apart from the sesame white and black seeds.

5. Then combine the miso dressing and sour cherries by hand and stir to combine.

6. To serve, use the sesame seeds for garnish.

Basil Cucumber Salad

Servings: 2

Ingredients

¼ cup fresh basil, chopped

½ red onion, diced small

2 cups cauliflower, chopped

1 English cucumber, quartered

For creamy lemon dressing

1 teaspoon Dijon mustard

1 teaspoon pure maple syrup

2 tablespoons plain hummus

Juice from 1 lemon

Extra chopped basil

Sea salt, to taste

Directions

1. Add the cauliflower into a food processor and then blend to make it crumbly.

2. Pour into a large bowl and then add in basil, red onion and cucumber, and combine completely.

3. Now make the dressing; whisk these dressing ingredients in a bowl and mix then pour over your salad.

4. Toss to combine and then serve.

Cucumber and Red Onion Salad

Servings: 2

Ingredients

Salt to taste

Juice of 1 fresh lime

¼ cup chopped fresh cilantro

1 large red onion, chopped

2 large cucumbers, peeled and sliced

4 tomatoes, chopped to 8 wedges

Directions

1. Combine the lime juice, cilantro, red onion, cucumbers, and tomatoes in a bowl.

2. Season with salt then serve.

Spring Green Salad

Servings: 4

Ingredients

½ cup raw pistachios

3 scallions, sliced

2 cups asparagus, sliced 1-inch pieces

3 kiwi, thinly sliced

2 large pears, thinly sliced

1 large bunch of kale, chopped

For dressing

Sea salt

1 tablespoon maple syrup

Zest of one lemon

3 tablespoons fresh lemon juice

3 tablespoons raw hemp oil

Directions

1. Into a large bowl, pour in the chopped kales. In another bowl, mix the dressing ingredients in a bowl.

2. Add in the dressing ingredients into the bowl with kales and massage the dressing into the chopped kales until it's well coasted and soft.

3. Now add in the other ingredients and toss to combine. Serve and enjoy.

Blueberry mango salad with tahini dressing

Servings: 1

Ingredients

¼ cup organic pecans

½ cup organic mango, cubed

½ cup organic blueberries

2 handfuls organic spring salad mix

Tahini ginger dressing

2 tablespoons filtered water

1/8 teaspoon ground ginger

½ tablespoon raw honey

2 tablespoons raw tahini

Directions

1. Onto a plate, place 2 handfuls of spring salad and then sprinkle in the blue berries, the mangos, and the pecans at the top.

2. To make the dressing, put all the dressing ingredients into a bowl then stir until well mixed. Adjust water if you like a thinner consistency.

3.Drizzle the dressing over the salad and serve.

Thai Coleslaw

Servings: 4

Ingredients

2 tablespoons honey or agave nectar

Himalaya sea salt

1 handful torn basil leafs

1 handful cilantro leafs

1 ripe mango cut in small dices

¼ cup carrots, shredded

¼ cup red cabbage, shredded

½ head white cabbage, shredded

1 cup raw almond or peanut butter

1 ½ tablespoons tamari

½ tablespoon red chili

2 tablespoons ginger, chopped

½ cup lemon juice

½ cup raw cashews

Directions

1. Begin by cutting the mango into little pieces and then shred the carrots and cabbages.

2. Process the red chili, ginger, lemon juice, and the honey in a high speed blender.

3. Add in the raw almond butter and continue to blend at low speed to mix. Continue until you obtain a thick cake batter-like mixture, which you can thin with a little water.

4. Combine the raw almond butter and the cabbage in a bowl and then add in mango pieces and raw cashews.

5. To top, use basil and cilantro leaves and few mango pieces or carrots for additional color.

Soup Recipes

Avocado Lime Soup

Servings: 3-4

Ingredients

Soup

1 cup water

1 teaspoon tamari

½ teaspoon salt

1 teaspoon coriander, ground

2 teaspoons cumin

Small handful of cilantro, fresh

Juice of 1 lime

1 stalk celery

¾ of a cucumber, medium-sized

2 avocados

For Sour cream

½ teaspoon salt

1 cup water

1 ½ tablespoons apple cider vinegar

2 tablespoons lemon juice

1 ½ cups cashew

Directions

1. To prepare the soup, blend the ingredients for soup in a high-speed blender.

2. Once smooth, pour into a serving bowl.

3. Prepare the sour cream by processing the ingredients in a high-speed blender. Then add in a little water at a time to make it easier to blend the cashews until smooth.

4. Pour the sour cream onto the smooth and enjoy.

Creamy Zucchini & Celery Soup

Servings: 4

Ingredients

1 cup filtered water

1 stalk celery, finely chopped

1 teaspoon garlic powder

2 tablespoons flax seed oil

1 avocado, chopped

1 teaspoon Himalayan crystal salt

2 tablespoons lemon juice

2 zucchini, chopped

1 tablespoon white miso paste

2 tablespoons fresh dill

½ celeriac, chopped

¼ white onion, chopped

Smoked paprika & fresh herbs to garnish

Directions

1. Into a high speed blender, mix all the ingredients and then add a cup of filtered water or more for desired consistency or taste.

2. Pour the soup into bowls and garnish with the smoked paprika alongside a sprinkle of fresh herbs.

Green Soup

Servings: 4

Ingredients

¼ cup raw cashews, soaked for 1-3 hours

1- 1½ cups water

1 lime or lemon, juiced

1 jalapeño pepper, seeded & cored

2 tablespoons chopped sweet onion

1 avocado

½ cucumber, peeled

1 zucchini, coarsely chopped

¼ cup parsley

¼ cup cilantro

2 stalks celery

2 cups spinach, loosely packed

½ teaspoon Himalayan sea salt

Garnish: chopped vegetables, hemp seeds or dulse flakes

Dash of black pepper

Directions

1. Into a food processor, blend spinach and then add a cup of water.

2. Add in the other ingredients and continue to process until you have a smooth and creamy mixture.

3. Serve the soup instantly or keep in the fridge for an hour. In case you don't prefer nuts, try substituting the cashews with more avocados.

Garlic Almond Soup

Servings: 1

Ingredients

½ teaspoon apple cider vinegar

1 tablespoon extra virgin olive oil

White pepper, to taste

Sea salt to taste

3 garlic cloves, finely grated

1½ cups almond milk, cold

To serve: freshly ground black pepper, olive oil, croutons, fresh coriander, lime

Directions

1. Put all the ingredients except those to be used in serving into a food processor or blender and then pulse until well combined.

2. Season with more salt and pepper if required and then serve. You can top with black pepper and lime juice, croutons

or raw cracker crumbles or with olive oil. Store the soup into the fridge to serve later.

Carrot Ginger Soup

Servings: 2-3

Ingredients

¼ teaspoon allspice

½ teaspoon ginger, chopped

½ teaspoons sea salt

Juice from ½ lemon

1 avocado

Juice from 1 green apple and 10 carrots

Directions

1. Place all the ingredients into a high-speed blender, and process until thick and smooth.

2. Serve and enjoy.

Cream of Spinach Soup

Servings: 2-4

Ingredients

Dash of nutmeg

Sea salt to taste

2 tablespoons lemon juice

½ cup cashews

1 cup cucumber juice

2 cups spinach

Directions

1. Process the ingredients to obtain a thick and smooth mixture.

2. Serve at room temperature.

Pasta And Noodle Recipes

Raw Pasta

Zucchini Pasta with cucumber and avocado sauce

Servings: 4

Ingredients

Arugula

Jalapeno, thinly sliced, without seeds

Mini heirloom tomatoes, grape or cherry, halved

4 large zucchini

Zest of 1 lemon

Pea shoots

For Cucumber-Avocado Puree

¼ teaspoon pepper

2 garlic cloves

1 lemon

Large basil leaves

1 cucumber, peeled and sliced thick

1 medium avocado

Salt to taste

Directions

1. Prepare zucchini noodles spiralized or julienne style.

2. To prepare the avocado puree, put the sauce ingredients into a blender and process until creamy.

3. Toss the avocado-cucumber puree with the zucchini pasta and a handful of arugula.

4. Now serve this with tomatoes, fresh cracked pepper, lemon wedges, lemon zest, jalapenos and peas shoots.

Spaghetti and Meatballs

Servings: 2-4

Ingredients

2-4 yellow and green zucchini cut on a spiral slicer and tossed with some lemon juice

For sauce

1 teaspoon sea salt

1 teaspoon Italian seasoning

1 handful fresh basil

1 pinch fresh oregano

3 tablespoons fresh parsley

2 cloves garlic

3 tablespoons olive oil

2 dates, soaked for 2 hrs

1 teaspoon tomato concentrate

1 cup sun dried tomatoes, soaked for 1-2 hrs

2 cups cherry tomatoes

For savory nut balls

2 teaspoons dried cilantro or 1-2 cups fresh

1 teaspoon cumin

Pinch of turmeric

1 sticks celery, minced

2 cloves garlic

¼ cup walnuts

½ cup sunflower seeds, soaked

1 cup almonds, soaked

1 cup burdock puree

2 carrots

1 bell pepper

1 small red onion

Directions

1. Start by processing the sauce ingredients in a high-speed blender until smooth. To make the sauce thinner, add tomato soak water.

2. To make the savory nut balls, blend the ingredients in a food processor and add in some water if required.

3. On the table, lay a parchment paper and place the nut ball mixture on it, and then position a second parchment paper on the mixture.

4. Now roll the dough into ½ inch thickness using your hand or with a rolling pin. Then cut out patty shapes using a cookie cutter or a cup and position the patties on Teflex sheets.

5. Dehydrate the patties at 145 degrees for 2 hours inside the Excalibur Dehydrator, then lower the temperature to 115 and continue with dehydration. Serve the sauce with savory nut balls and zucchini after achieving the preferred consistency.

Noodle Recipes

Kelp Noodles with Spicy Peanut Sauce

Servings: 4

Ingredients

1 cup organic red bell peppers, chopped

1 cup organic spinach, diced

12-ounce Packet Sea tangle Kelp Noodles

For Sauce

1 teaspoon Himalayan pink salt

1 organic jalapeno

2 cloves organic garlic, crushed

1 tablespoon organic cilantro

2 tablespoons organic extra-virgin olive oil

3 tablespoons organic raw coconut crystals

½ cup peanut butter, organic

1 can organic full-fat coconut milk or homemade raw milk

1 teaspoon organic red pepper flakes

Directions

1. Start by preparing the kelp noodles: just take them out of the package, rinse them using clean filtered water and then set it aside.

2. To prepare the veggies, chop the spinach into thin strips followed by the red bell peppers and set them aside.

3. Now make the sauce by combining all sauce ingredients into a powerful blender. Blend the ingredients until you obtain a creamy and soft consistency.

4. Adjust the seasonings, as you prefer, particularly the red pepper flakes and the jalapeno. It's okay to add in about ¼-½ cup of filtered water to create a thinner sauce.

5. Into a medium sized bowl, put the chopped spinach, kelp noodles and then pour the sauce ingredients over the top. Stir gently to distribute the contents.

6. If desired, you can garnish with red bell pepper strips or extra chopped spinach.

Zucchini noodles with pumpkin Seed and Arugula Pesto

Servings: 4

Ingredients

4 Zucchini, julienned

½ cup olive oil

2 tablespoons nutritional yeast

2 medium peeled garlic cloves, chopped

2 tablespoons fresh parsley, chopped

1 cup arugula leaves, packed

1 cup basil leaves, packed

1 ½ teaspoons sea salt

2 tablespoons fresh lemon juice

½ cup raw pumpkin seeds

Directions

1. Mix the nutritional yeast, garlic, parsley, arugula, basil, sea salt and lemon juice in a blender.

2. Process the ingredients until smooth and then add in a little olive oil. Continue to blend until it's well incorporated.

3. Add in some pumpkin seeds and continue to blend to smoothness.

4. To serve, toss with zucchini noodles.

Lemon Herb Noodles

Servings: 2-3

Ingredients

Kelp noodles

For the cheese sauce

Pinch of salt

1 tablespoon water

1 tablespoon olive oil

2 sprigs rosemary

1 tablespoon parsley

1 green onion, thinly sliced

1 tablespoon nutritional yeast

½ teaspoon soy sauce

1 ½ teaspoons lemon zest

Juice of 1 lemon

1 cup cashews, soaked for 2 hours

Micro-greens and chopped parsley

Directions

1. Put all the ingredients for the cheese sauce in a high-speed blender and process until smooth and thick. Add some lemon juice or water if the sauce is too thick.

2. Keep the noodles in a zip lock baggie that is completely sealed and place in a warm water bath in order to keep them warm.

3. Mix the sauce and noodles and stir well, then garnish with lemon zest, micro-greens and parsley.

Other Dinner Recipes

Zucchini nest lasagna

Servings: 2

Ingredients

¼ cup whole raw organic cashews, ground

½ cup raw cashew cheese

2 tablespoons fresh organic garlic, finely chopped

½ cup fresh organic basil, finely chopped

1 teaspoon raw apple cider vinegar, organic

2 tablespoons raw organic coconut aminos

¼ cup fresh organic oregano leaves, packed

6 large garlic cloves, fresh and organic

6 small vine ripe tomatoes, organic

4 fresh organic zucchinis, medium-sized

Raw cashew cheese

1/3 cup water

1 small ripe lemon

¼ cup raw organic apple cider vinegar

2 cups whole raw organic cashews

Directions

1. Pulse the apple cider vinegar, coconut aminos, oregano leaves, 6 cloves of garlic and tomatoes in a food processor.

2. Place the mixture onto a dehydrator for 8 hours ensuring to stir each hour to create your tomato sauce. One hour before complete dehydration of tomato sauce, mix garlic and chopped basil in a small bowl and set aside.

3. Hold the nub end of the zucchini flat onto a cutting board and then use a vegetable peeler to make ribbons from the nub to the other end. Continue to make the ribbons on one side until halfway. Flip and make ribbons on the other side as well.

4. Put the zucchini ribbons onto different piles and use a standard glass shot to wrap a ribbon around the glass at the mouth, placed on the cutting board. Pick the next zucchini ribbon, and wrap it about ½-inch overlapping the initial ribbon and progress all around the glass. Layer the other ribbons up until when 2/3 of the ribbons are used.

5. Take out the glass shot gently to obtain the outer ring of the zucchini nest. Use the ribbons that remain to fill the hole of the nest into X-shapes using ribbon halves, to make a cup

without holes. Do the operation with the entire zucchini sets to make 4 nests.

6. Quarter the cashew cheese to form 4 balls and roll the balls into the garlic and basil mixture to completely coat all sides. Put 1 herbed ball into the nest and then pat down gently, and process with the other pieces.

7. Put the flat drips rack into the bottom of a large casserole dish and then position the filled nests into the middle of the large piece of tin foil in rows of 2 and then seal it. To seal, just make a pouch for them but don't squish.

8. Then position the pouch onto the drip rack and fill the bottom of your casserole dish. Ensure to cover the bottom about 1/2-inch of the tin foil pouch with hot water at 116 degrees.

9. Use the tin foil to cover the entire pan and allow to set for about 20 minutes into the 116 degree water. You can then remove the pouch from the rack very carefully.

10. To serve, plate each of your nests using a ¼ of the tomato sauce and use a ¼ of the cashews for garnish. Enjoy your zucchini nest lasagna.

Directions for raw cashew cheese

1. Break the cashews into quarters in a large bowl then soak the cashew pieces in clean water for around 16 hours. Drain

the cashews and rinse well then blend the cashews with lemon juice and vinegar in a high-speed blender. Add a tablespoon of water at a time to make the cheese smooth.

2. Open up several cheesecloths and layer on each other then spoon the cheese and put in the center then gather the sides of cheesecloths in order to make a pouch then twist and tie the top and tie using a rubber band then hang it and allow to drain.

3. Suspend the cheese ball over a container to allow it to drain ensuring that the container is at least 2 inches deeper than the cheese ball. Hang for 24 hours then unwrap the cheese gently and set aside.

Raw Pizza Extravaganza

Servings: 4

Ingredients

Crust

½ cup fresh basil

pinch Celtic sea salt

1 cup cashews

For tomato sauce

1 tablespoon honey

1 cup sundried tomatoes

Cheese

1 tablespoon water

1 clove garlic, with core removed

½ cup fresh basil

Celtic sea salt

Juice of ½ lemon

1 cup cashews, soaked 6-12 hours

Toppings

½ cup button mushrooms, thinly sliced

1 stick celery, thinly sliced

½ red bell pepper, finely chopped

1 yellow tomato, cubed

1 tablespoon chopped black olives, seed removed

½ cup cilantro, chopped finely

For Marinade

1 teaspoon honey

Pinch of salt

1 tablespoon water

1 tablespoon olive oil

½ lemon, juiced

Directions

1. To marinate toppings mix all the topping ingredients in a bowl. Add in the marinade ingredients and allow time to marinate as you prepare the other pizza ingredients. To make the softest topping, put the marinade into a glass bowl outside in the sun for few hours, with a glass lid on.

2. To make the crust, just blend the cup of cashews into fine powder and also blend the salt and basil. Mix with your hands and then pour into a round crust on a plate. Once done with the shaping of the crust, loosen the crust with a spatula from the bottom of the plate.

3. Prepare the tomato sauce by blending the ingredients to obtain a smooth mixture. Then pour your sauce onto the pizza crust and smooth it out to completely cover the crust.

4. Then make the cheese by processing its ingredients into a creamy sauce, and pour onto the tomato sauce. Smooth the cheese sauce evenly.

5. Finally pour the toppings on the pizza, slice and serve.

Raw Taco shells with fillings

Yields 30-40 small taco shells

Ingredients

Taco Shells

Celtic sea salt to taste

2 tablespoons poppy seeds

1 teaspoon cumin powder

1 teaspoon cayenne powder

1 teaspoon chili powder

3 teaspoons minced garlic, with skin

2 tablespoon sweet onion, minced

1 cup sprouted sunflower seeds

1 cup brown flax seeds, finely ground

2 cups golden flax seeds, finely ground

For Guacamole Salsa

1-2 pinch Celtic sea salt

1 teaspoons cayenne powder

½ clove minced garlic

1 tablespoon lemon or lime juice

4 tablespoons parsley, cilantro and marjoram, chopped

1 tablespoons red onion, minced

1 avocado, diced

For Sour Cream

4 tablespoons of fresh herbs, chopped

¾ cup water

2 pinches of Celtic sea salt

2 tablespoons lemon juice

½ cup pine nuts

1 cup raw cashews, soaked for 4 hrs

Mango Salsa

1 tablespoon red onion, minced

½ teaspoon Celtic sea salt

2 tablespoons lime or lemon juice

4 tablespoons cilantro, chopped

1 tablespoon fresh hot pepper, minced

 2 ripe mangoes, peeled, cut 1/4 inch cubes

"Refried Beans"

Celtic sea salt

1-2 dates

1 teaspoon cumin powder

1 teaspoon cayenne or 2 teaspoons chili powder

3 teaspoons sweet onion, minced

2 teaspoons lemon juice

1 clove fresh garlic, with skin

3 tablespoons sesame seed butter

1 cup sunflower seeds, sprouted

Directions

1. Prepare the taco shells by combing the ingredients in a blender until smooth. To constitute a batter-like consistency, add some water and continue to blend until smooth. Then keep the batter in the fridge for around 8-12 hours.

2. Place a thin layer of the taco batter using a spatula onto a Teflex sheets, and then dehydrate for 3-5 hours at 105 degrees F. Once done, remove from the sheets and use a cookie cutter to cut out rounds from the dough.

3. Place the cut out rounds and keep them into the dehydrator for 2 hours on Teflex sheets at similar temperature.

4. Once done, remove the taco shells and now fold them onto each other to create a taco shell. Put them back into the dehydrator shelves for around 10-12 hours to firm up into crisps.

5. Make the Guacamole Salsa ingredients

6. Prepare the sour cream by blending the ingredients in a high-speed blender to a thick and smooth consistency.

7. For mad mango salsa, just toss the ingredients together in a bowl and serve.

8. Now process the ingredients for refried beans in a food processor until smooth; then add in salt or additional spices if needed.

9. To serve, pick the crisp taco shell and then spoon 1-2 tablespoons of refried beans or salsa into the shell. You can also top with bell peppers, cucumber, sliced tomatoes or lettuce. Eat it immediately.

Shiitake, Avocado, and Pickled Ginger Sushi Rolls

Makes 6-8 rolls

Ingredients

For Filling

½ cup beet juice

¾ cup agave nectar

1 ½ cups raw apple cider vinegar, or rice wine vinegar

2 tablespoons sea salt

2 large young ginger-roots, sliced on a mandolin

2 tablespoons extra-virgin olive oil

¾ cup nama shoyu

1 cup shiitake mushroom caps, thinly sliced

For Rice

3 tablespoons agave nectar

¼ cup brown rice wine vinegar

2 teaspoons sea salt

½ cup pine nuts

6 cups chopped jicama

For Assembly

2 tablespoons black sesame seeds

½ cup wasabi

2 green onions, white and 1 inch of green, sliced

1 small bunch sunflower sprouts

2 ripe avocados, pitted, and sliced

1 medium cucumber, seeded, and thinly julienned

6 to 8 sheets nori, un-toasted

Directions

1. To make the filling, toss the mushrooms with olive oil and ¼ cup Nama shoyu. Let it marinate for an hour before you drain and set aside.

2. Into a bowl, put sliced ginger and add salt. After 5 minutes, rinse, drain and squeeze out water.

3. Put 2/3 of ginger into a bowl plus ½ cup agave nectar and a cup of vinegar. Put remaining vinegar and agave into a small bowl and then julienne the ginger that remains.

4. Add in juice to julienned ginger that is completely immersed in agave and vinegar liquid. Cover the bowls and keep in the fridge for 1-3 days. Later, drain well to use.

5. For rice, put the pine nuts and jicama into a blender and pulse to obtain rice-sized grains. Then press the jicama on clean paper or kitchen towels to remove moisture.

6. Mix together agave nectar, rice vinegar, rice and salt and then spread this mixture onto a dehydrator for 2 hours at 115 degrees F to eliminate moisture.

7. Occasionally toss the rice to prevent over-drying and turning pale brown. Otherwise add some seasoning liquid if this happens.

8. For assembly, put the nori sheet on a bamboo mat, with the rough side up. Ensure the short side is facing you, the sheet being in portrait mode.

9. Put ½ cup of rice on the sheet of nori, spread it evenly to about bottom 1/3rd of the sheet, but with an inch allowance on the bottom. Lay some julienned ginger, sprouts, shiitake filling, avocados and cucumber across the rice.

10. Sprinkle with green onion and spread wasabi across the exposed nori before you roll it. It's easier to spread wasabi on nori compared to distributing evenly with the other filling.

11. Now fold the bottom of the bamboo mat and over your filling and then roll the nori firmly. Then use some water to wet the top edge of the nori to assist in sealing it shut.

12. Press the roll in the mat for some time to allow it set and seal completely. Unwrap the meat gently and then cut your rolls into 6 pieces using a sharp knife.

13. With a wet towel placed between cuts, begin by cutting the rolls into half, and then each half into 3 evenly sized pieces to get 6 pieces.

14. Finally position the sushi onto a plate and then sprinkle with sesame seeds. To garnish, use some bits of wasabi or a little pile of pickled ginger slices.

Raw Pate & Collard Wrap

Ingredients

A few drops of extra virgin olive oil

Pinch of curry

Pinch of cumin

Pinch of sea salt

3-4 soaked sundried tomatoes

1 cup celery, chopped

1 cup carrots, chopped

1 cup walnuts

1 bunch collard greens

Directions

1. Into a high-speed blender, put the above ingredients except the collard greens and then blend to create a pate consistency.

2. Pour the pate into the collard greens then wrap.

Stuffed Kale Leaves with Cashew Aioli

Servings: 4

Ingredients

Bunch of kale leaves

For the stuffing

½ cup organic raisins, diced

2 cups organic fresh mint, minced

1 cup organic sun-dried tomatoes, diced

5 sprigs green onions, organic

1 teaspoon pink Himalayan salt

2 tablespoons lemon juice, organic

½ teaspoon cinnamon, organic

3 teaspoons lemon zest

½ cup pine nuts

1 clove garlic

½ cup organic olive oil

3 cups raw cauliflower, organic

For the aioli

1/3 cup organic mint leaves, tightly packed

½ cup purified or distilled water

5 cloves garlic

1 teaspoon lemon zest

½ teaspoon raw honey or organic raw agave nectar

½ teaspoon pink Himalayan salt

1 ¼ tablespoons organic lemon juice

1 cup organic cashews

Directions

1. To prepare the stuffing, first put the parsnip or cauliflower into a blender and pulse it to achieve a rice-like appearance. Then put the pulsed rice into a large bowl, and set it aside.

2. Into a high speed blender, add in all the stuffing ingredients apart from the sun-dried tomatoes, raisins and mint leaves.

3. Process into creamy consistency and add the mixture to the rice, and then combine using your hand.

4. Now add in the sundried tomatoes, the raisins and mint leaves to this mixture and mix using your hand.

5. To make the aioli, combine the ingredients in a blender and process until creamy. Transfer the contents into a bowl, and add in the diced mint leaves by hand.

6. Obtain a piece of kale leaf and remove the bottom part of the stem, which can be used to juice.

7. Then spread about 1-2 tablespoons of the stuffing mix onto a kale leaf using a spatula and then roll them up.

8. Once done, serve with the aioli and enjoy.

Raw French Fries

Servings: 2

Ingredients

1 teaspoon sea salt

2 teaspoons curcumin

½ cup olive or hemp seed oil, cold pressed

4 kohlrabis

For Ketchup

½ cup pure water

1 squeeze lemon juice

5 dates

3 pieces sun dried tomatoes

3 tomatoes

Directions

1. Begin by cutting the kohlrabis cabbage just like French fries and then put in a bowl.

2. Put some salt, curcumin and oil into a bowl and combine; and then pour this mixture over your fries.

3. Allow the mixture to chill for around 10 minutes, and then drain.

4. Scoop the mixture into paper towels to remove any excess oil.

5. To prepare the ketchup, place the ingredients in a powerful blender starting with water, lemon juice and tomatoes. Put the dried tomatoes and the dates on top and blend completely. Serve the French fries with the ketchup.

Cauliflower rice

Servings: 2

Ingredients

Pink Himalayan salt

Extra virgin olive oil

Apple cider vinegar

3-4 tablespoons of nutritional yeast flakes

1 large cauliflower

Directions

1. Start by grating the cauliflower and combine it with the nutritional yeast flakes. Then use the apple cider vinegar to season, and then add some salt and olive oil.

2. To make the cauliflower sweet, add in lemon juice in place of apple cider vinegar alongside cardamom, ground cinnamon, lemon zest and some currants. Also try sweetening with some raw agave nectar or raw honey.

3. For sweet and sour taste, just add in dries barberries, ground sumac and raw agave nectar. Include a small piece of fresh pineapple if desired.

4. Try other tastes such as Italian green by adding marjoram, rosemary, thyme, oregano and basil, or Thai green by adding finely chopped methi leaves and cilantro.

5. Try adding tarragon, parsley and finely chopped dill for fresh green taste or season with ground cumin, ground pepper peppercorns and paprika for Hungarian taste.

Raw Tagliatelle with Mushroom and Walnut Sauce

Servings: 4

Ingredients

1 garlic clove

1 tablespoon zucchini, blended

2-3 tablespoons water

2-3 tablespoons extra virgin olive oil

1 small Jerusalem artichoke

2 tablespoons walnuts

2 tablespoons porcini mushrooms, dried

4-5 zucchini

Saffron

Fresh parsley

Fresh rosemary

Black pepper

Celtic salt

Directions

1. First soak the dried mushrooms in water for 24 hours, drain and later toss into marinade consisting of chopped garlic, rosemary, parsley, pepper, salt and a tablespoon of

olive oil. Allow the mushroom to marinate overnight, then discard the garlic.

2. To make the sauce, just toss the other ingredients apart from the saffron and zucchini into a food processor. Process them to obtain a coarsely blended mixture, ensuring to scrap down the blender jar occasionally. Then put this in the fridge for some time.

3. Peel the zucchini before cutting them down using a mandolin or potato peeler into tagliatelle.

4. Set the zucchini into a colander, add in salt and allow to drip for around 30 minutes, and then wrap them in a kitchen paper. Ensure that you squeeze to get rid of water.

5. Now transfer the zucchini into a bowl, add in the saffron powder and combine to get a homogeneous color.

6. To serve, top the tagliatelle with walnut halves alongside parsley sprinkle.

Raw artichoke and Spinach Sauce

Servings: 2

Ingredients

100 g fresh spinach leaves

4 Jerusalem artichokes

50 g raw cashews

Extra virgin olive oil

Nutmeg, freshly grated

Pink pepper, freshly ground

Himalayan salt

Water

Garnish: dehydrated onions and pink pepper grains

Directions

1. Soak the cashews in water overnight, then drain and rinse them.

2. Scrub, peel and chop the artichokes then wash the spinach.

3. Into a blender, place the spinach, artichokes and the cashews alongside nutmeg, pepper, salt and water and process on high speed.

4. Once smooth and warm, garnish with olive oil, pink pepper grains and dehydrated onions.

Conclusion

Thank you again for downloading this book!

Most people frown upon a raw food diet thinking that they will only be taking fruits and vegetables. However, as you have seen from the above recipes, embracing a raw food diet does not mean that you will only be eating vegetables but as you can see, you can still enjoy your oats, some amazing cereals, pancakes, bread and even cupcakes.

Start by shopping for all the groceries you would need and don't fall into the temptation of unhealthy eating habits. It is also important to start slow. For instance, you can start by changing your breakfast to raw food then over time change your lunch and dinner. This is likely to be much easier as compared to cutting cold turkey.

I hope this book has provided you adequate information about starting on a raw food diet and what to watch out for.

The next step is to first consult your doctor to know that it is safe to start on a raw diet, then you can start buying the foods you want for a healthy start.

Finally, if you enjoyed this book, would you be kind enough to leave a review for this book on Amazon?

Click here to leave a review for this book on Amazon!

Thank you and good luck!

RAW FOOD

www.ingramcontent.com/pod-product-compliance
Lightning Source LLC
Chambersburg PA
CBHW031153020426
42333CB00013B/640